The
Smart Shred
Diet

A Customised Nutrition Plan To Get Chiselled Abs Without Cutting Out Your Favourite Foods

TOMMY COLE MSc

Disclaimer

This book is not intended for the treatment or prevention of disease, nor as a substitute for medical treatment, nor as an alternative to medical advice. Use of the guidelines herein is at the sole choice and risk of the reader.

Copyright: © 2018 by Thomas Cole. All rights reserved.

No part of The Smart Shred Diet may be reproduced or transmitted in any form whatsoever, electronic or mechanical, including photocopying recording, or by any informational storage or retrieval system, without expressed, written and signed permission from the author (with the exception of brief quotations as used in reviews or discussion groups, with attribution to the author and source).

For information contact: tommy@tommycole.co.uk

Acknowledgements

A big thanks goes to the coffees and country music that fuelled the writing of this book; without them, the hours of keypad pushing wouldn't have been possible.

On a serious note, a huge thank you goes to everyone who helped me produce this book, with particular thanks going to Richie, Troy, and Richard.

Table Of Contents

Foreword

Nutrition, fitness, health, dieting, the gym – it's confusing right? It is, if you listen to the wrong people. When people are surveyed on health and fitness the #1 complaint that gets quoted is people find it confusing: "He said this, she said that, this magazine said its bad for you, that research said it's good for you, they had a debate and no one could decide what was correct, it's just so hard to know fact from fiction".

In this conundrum there is responsibility on both sides of the fence. The fitness industry, us, needs to be more responsible with the information it puts out (advice based on science, not blogs we've read from people with good abs), and the people reading it and making plans for their health and fitness need to have a finely tuned BS radar that knows how to filter fact from fiction (not follow what Dave down the pub said, or OK Magazine).

As I write this foreword "Skinny Jabs" has just hit the weight loss market – that's a jab that cost £200 and helps you lose weight. Except it doesn't, well, it does if you follow a Calorie controlled diet and exercise. Shock horror. This is a mad reflection on the ethics of the health and fitness industry, but also a reflection on how most people's mindsets work. Everyone's looking for the quick fix, the silver bullet, the way they can get all the results with none of the effort.

Well I'll be the bearer of bad news. The silver bullet doesn't exist. As I write this foreword I am 32 years of age, and at the age of 18 I started my weight loss and health journey. At the time I was obese and suffered with ADHD, Eczema, Asthma, and IBS. I lost all the weight by eating better, hitting the gym, and I solved all my health issues by spending time working through all the different processes and therapies that help such issues. I did the work, and so will you have to do the work.

Please don't see this as a negative, see it as a positive. 14 years later I am still learning, evolving, tweaking, and enjoying mastering my health and fitness, trying to find better ways of doing things, and generally living what I describe as "an awesome life". The good thing is, you're in good hands. I've been there and done it, and the man that has written this book has equally put in the work to earn his personal stripes to empower others, adding to that his credibility.

I first met Tommy Cole in our education programs – I run a nutrition education company called The BTN Academy and Tommy was a student – so he studied under me and loads of amazing tutors. Tommy then progressed into more advanced learning, including 2 nutrition master's that focused on studying the intricacies of human health and performance. He became a coach, helping 1000s of people to reclaim their health and develop bullet-proof fitness.

If you want someone to trust, trust this book and trust Tommy. This book is full of rational, realistic, honest, evidence based advice on how to get fit, be healthy and happy, and become a high performing human that looks awesome. You can trust this book because Tommy has made it his mission to become trustworthy and teach the right thing. In developing your knowledge from this book you'll then develop your BS radar – you'll start to see the fads, and you'll start to see the light.

Now, while this book speaks sense, you still have to do the work, be willing to change and explore new possibilities for your body and mind. Don't see this as a negative thing. See this as an opportunity and embark on your health and fitness journey today. It changed my life, it changed Tommy's life, and it can change yours.

Ben Coomber

Who is Ben Coomber?

Ben is a Performance Nutritionist (CISSN), coach (S&C), international speaker, and fitness educator. Ben has the UK's #1 rated Health and Fitness podcast, Ben Coomber Radio, has coached 1000s of people in his 90 day program Fat Loss for Life, has consulted and worked with everyone from pro athletes to kids playing sport, educates the nutrition coaches of the future at The BTN Academy, owns Awesome Supplements, has worked with companies like Sky TV, O2, and Twinnings Tea, has been a headline speaker at Body Power, SFN, and Be Fit for many years, and continues to try to educate and innovate in the world of fitness. This all stemmed from his journey as an obese teenager wanting to better his health, body, and mind.

About The Author

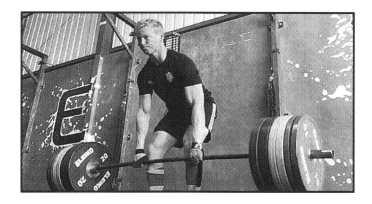

Hi,

I'm Tommy; I like bicep curls, coffee, and cake.

When I'm not at the gym, or having coffee and cake, I like to bury my head in nutritional science, learning all there is to know about building a chiselled body with rippling abs. In fact, I'm such a nutrition nerd that I've completed two nutrition master's degrees to quench my thirst for knowledge. Pretty ~~lame~~ damn fricken cool, right?

This book has been a natural result of my years of training, studying, and experience gained helping people achieve their body transformation goals.

I hope you enjoy it, and I am confident that you'll see great results if you apply its contents.

Big love,

Tommy – your favourite, blonde haired, polar bear complexioned nutritionist.

PREFACE

You know those beat-around-the-bush type books that seem to spend a lifetime before getting to the point? Well, this isn't going to be one of them. I mean, I could babble on for days about the intricacies of protein synthesis, metabolism, and digestion, but to you that would make this book just about as dull as a vegetarian sausage at a steakhouse.

So, in this book, I'll be steering clear of the irrelevant junk and instead, I'll be sharing with you all you need to know to become a fat loss ninja and ultimately, reveal your cheese grater like abs.

Because I get that many people are like me and have the attention span of a goldfish, the chapters are kept short, the key points are summarised at the end of each, and I've included "The 10 Commandments Of The Smart Shred Diet" in Chapter 15 to give an extremely concise breakdown of the book's main recommendations. Feel free to skip to the key points, and Chapter 15, if you're in a rush to get started, but I highly recommend you read the book in its entirety.

You Know What's Also Cool About This Book?

Well, unlike most popular diet/nutrition books that are simply based on what the current trend is, all the guidance this one provides is backed up by a shed load of scientific evidence and knowledge which I've acquired through thousands of hours spent studying nutrition, and applying it to myself and clients.

I've compiled a reference list of the scientific studies this book has evolved from, as well as some recommended reading and watching, which you can find in the book's bonus content area if you're keen to take your knowledge one step further. You'll also find copies of all the book's tables, figures, and example diet and training plans there. I refer to some of this bonus material throughout the book, and you can unlock it at the following link by using the password: doughnut

www.tommycole.co.uk/bookbonuscontent

Anywhoo, that's enough rambling for one book; so let's get on with the important stuff now.

PART 1

THE SET UP

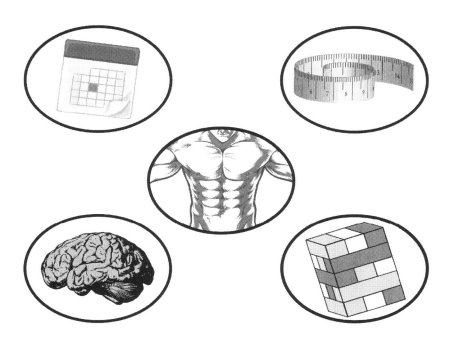

CHAPTER 1

The Reason You Need To Read This Book

I could barely move, my belly was ready to burst, and I lay on my bed in a pool of guilt, shame, and anger at myself after pigging out at a Chinese buffet in the midst of my fat loss diet.

While this might seem dramatic to some, if you've ever been dieting, only to fall off the wagon by going big on a cheat meal with no limits, I bet you're sat there nodding your head as you recount a similar experience.

Despite my discomfort, and the rollercoaster of emotion I felt, I found myself in the same situation every week: eating clean throughout the week, but then binging on everything I had restricted myself from on the weekend, leading to my physical and psychological discomfort.

Not only did this pattern make me feel like rubbish, but it put speed bumps on my road to the six pack I had always wanted.

In fact, by the time I eventually reached my goal weight and desired level of leanness (i.e. I had achieved the "Shred"), I was so fed up of dieting that I flipped the switch and ate like a ravaged pig, undoing much of my hard work and the countless weeks of restriction and dieting.

This left me deflated and in search of a better way to attain my dream physique: a strong, muscular body, with chiselled abs.

As a result of my search, I ended up becoming fascinated by

nutrition, which led me to study two master's degrees on the subject. Because of my personal experiences with dieting, much of my studying and research revolved around muscle gain and fat loss, and I became obsessed with finding the most effective ways to build a lean, and athletic, Herculean physique.

Ultimately, this led me to discover a number of dieting methods that challenged my beliefs, as they went completely against much of what I had always thought. I realised I didn't have to be as strict with my diet, that the conventional methods of dieting were the opposite of what I should be doing, and that eating the foods I loved every day would actually improve my results. In fact, scientific research had been showing all this for years!

Despite what the science says, fad diets still litter book shelves, celebrities continue to promote ineffective fat loss solutions, and many personal trainers advise clients to follow horrifically bland and repetitive diets that rarely lead to long term results. Consequently, dieters, just like you, have become confused by all the conflicting information and struggle to shred body fat more than ever before.

However, if everyone understood a few simple nutritional concepts and strategies (which I refer to as the "Smart"), then dieting and achieving a chiselled physique with rippling abs would be more effective, easier, and sustainable than ever. This scientific approach to fat loss I call "The Smart Shred Diet", and it is why this book is here. It will provide you with these concepts and strategies, meaning that you won't have to go through the same struggles most people do when dieting:

- You'll feel more in control of your diet and body.

- You'll no longer be confused by the conflicting messages in the media.

- You'll be able to enjoy your favourite foods while stripping body fat.

- You'll have the exact step by step process my clients and I have used to great success to get ripped abs and into the best shape of our lives.

It is for these reasons I've written this book and why it's so important for you to digest and apply its content (pun very much intended). By doing so, you'll achieve the "Smart", and "Shred" objectives of this book. The "Smart" refers to you gaining the nutrition knowledge required to become a fat loss ninja, and the "Shred" is the process of attaining a ripped body, which you'll be guided through, step by step.

So, if you're confused and frustrated by the contradictory advice about what you should eat, how much you should eat, and how to achieve and maintain a lean, athletic physique, make the commitment to both reading and applying the information in this book. If you do, you'll be making the all important first step to attaining a chiselled, athletic body, and won't have to starve, give up your favourite foods, or miss out on social occasions to do so.

Key Points

- The contents of this book will put an end to your dieting confusion.

- The objectives are to teach you exactly how to attain a ripped body (the "Smart"), and provide a step by step process to follow on your "Shred".

- By the end you'll know the exact steps to take to shred body fat fast and maintain your results.

CHAPTER 2

What Most People Don't Know About Nutrition: Nutritional Jenga

You know how a load of fitness gurus tell you to eat little and often, down a protein shake the second your foot leaves the gym floor, and avoid all sugary foods if you want to give yourself any chance of making progress?

Well, while they're not entirely wrong when they say these things can impact your results, they do often exaggerate their importance. So, this chapter is here to clear up the confusion.

To do that, I'm going to introduce to you a concept that shows how various nutritional variables differ in their importance when it comes to your physique. I call it "Nutritional Jenga",* and understanding the nutrition hierarchy it represents is vital to knowing how you should eat to get a ripped set of abs – most people don't know about it though.

At the foundation of the Nutritional Jenga tower, we have Calories, protein, and carbs/fat (see Figure 1). This signifies that they have the greatest bearing on your physique, because they're the most foundational to the tower's stability. At various points in this book I make reference to Calories, protein, carbs, and fat collectively as the "Foundation Blocks" of the tower.

If you've never heard of Jenga, it's a game where you start with a tower of rectangular blocks, and take it in turns to remove a block at a time until someone causes the tower to fall and consequently, loses.

In contrast to the Foundation Blocks, the other blocks/nutrition variables are far less important from a body transformation perspective, and they don't have to be dialled in to keep the tower standing (i.e. for you to see results). The less important variables I'm referring to here are your meal timing, meal frequency, and supplements: collectively they're called the "Minutia Blocks".

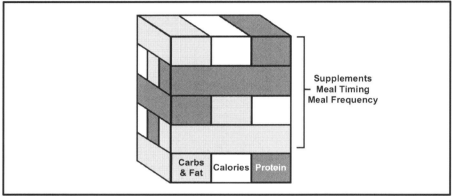

Figure 1.

FOUNDATION BLOCK 1 = CALORIES

Going deeper, Calories can be thought of as a lone block sitting slap bang in the centre of the tower's foundation. They can hold the tower up on their own, meaning that you will lose weight/fat if you get your Calorie intake right ONLY, regardless of any other nutritional variables. Getting your Calorie intake wrong is like moving the centre block, which will end up jeopardising the tower's stability, and making it topple over (synonymous to your results being non-existent).*

If you're a smart-arse, you might be thinking that the tower would also stand if the two blocks on the ends were supporting the tower only (the protein and carbs & fat blocks). The thing is, protein, carbs, and fat are where you get Calories from, so if you were to get your intake of them correct (i.e. get those blocks in place), then you would get your Calories right by default anyway.

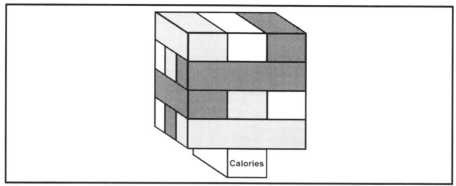

Figure 2.

FOUNDATION BLOCK 2 = PROTEIN

Next up is protein, which can be thought of as an additional block alongside Calories; it adds a great deal of stability to the single Calorie block on its own. This means that Calories and protein are the most important variables influencing your physique from a nutritional perspective.

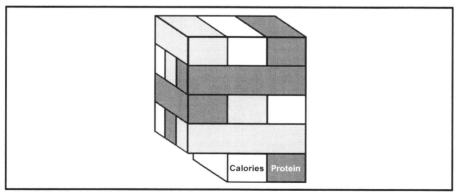

Figure 3.

FOUNDATION BLOCK 3 = CARBS AND FAT

The final Foundation Block is your carbohydrate and fat intake, which will add a further level of stability, but less relative to adding the protein block to Calories.

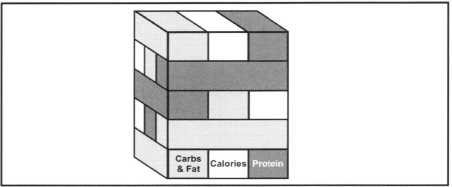

Figure 4.

THE OTHER BLOCKS AREN'T AS IMPORTANT

Meal frequency, meal timing, and supplements can also be important, but relative to the foundations of the tower, they won't have a big impact on your results.

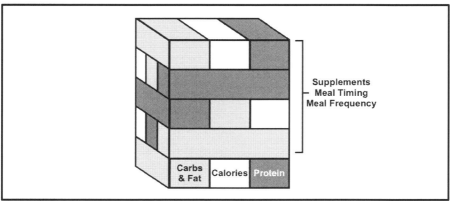

Figure 1.

So, you should prioritise getting your Calorie, protein, carb, and fat intake correct first, then start thinking more about how to dial in the minutia.

I know what you're thinking:

What About Food Quality? Surely An Apple Will Make You More Shredded Than A Slice Of Cake?

The issue with placing food quality in the Jenga tower is that it's hard to quantify its impact on your physique and fat loss, as it doesn't really have a direct impact like the other factors do.

For example, provided you consumed the correct number of Calories and macronutrients (protein, carbs, and fat), you would, most likely, end up with the same end beach bod whether getting them from peanut butter, protein shakes, and ice cream or from whole foods.

With that said, you're less likely to stick to your diet and eat the correct amount of Calories if all you eat is "junk" as it won't fill you up like whole foods would, and it would just make you feel like arse the whole time.

So food quality has an indirect effect on your physique by influencing the factors that have a direct effect, like Calories, and protein.

In fact, there are many other very important factors that can cause you to knock over your Nutritional Jenga tower; I call them Indirect Effecters.

Indirect Effecters Of Your Physique Transformation Represent Your Jenga Playing Strategy

Indirect Effecters involve your dietary mindset, food quality, and the approach you take to managing your diet.

More specifically, the Indirect Effecters are your:

- Goals

- Preferences

- Situation

- Nutrition knowledge

- Food choices

- Dietary management method

(Don't worry about remembering them all now).

These Indirect Effecters bring about changes to your physique by altering the Direct Effecters (Calories, protein etc), as represented in the flow chart below.

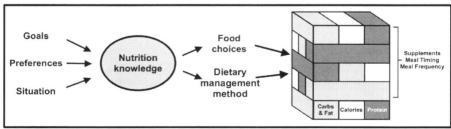

Figure 5.

As an example, your goal of losing fat (Goal) combined with your understanding that Calories are king of fat loss (Nutrition knowledge) may make you choose a low Calorie food (Food choice), which will contribute to the Direct Effecter of your overall daily intake of Calories.

So, in the Jenga analogy:

Think of the Indirect Effecters as your Jenga playing strategy, which is synonymous to your Nutrition Strategy.

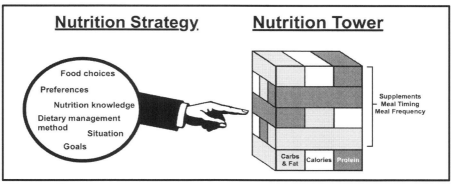

Figure 6.

If you suck or play stupid-arse moves (synonymous to eating lots of "junk", having an unrealistic goal, choosing a dietary management method that doesn't suit you, etc), you'll end up getting the Direct Effecters wrong, meaning you'll knock over your dietary tower. With that in mind, the key to a successful diet is correctly implementing the Indirect and Direct Effectors so they work together in unison.

For the rest of this book I'm going to be referring to Direct Effecters collectively as your Nutrition Tower, and Indirect Effecters as your Nutrition Strategy.

13

I get that this might sound a little confusing, but you don't need to grasp it all right now. The main point to take away is that there are lots of things that can impact your quest for abs. Fundamentally, your Nutrition Tower is what causes you to lose fat and transform your physique, but your Nutrition Strategy is just as important as it will change your physique via its impact on the blocks in the tower.

So, a successful diet requires you to become a Nutritional Jenga playing ninja by having a standing Nutrition Tower in the first place, and then playing the game strategically. The rest of this book will explain how to do this:

- *Part 1: The Set Up* – Defines your goals and expectations to ensure you start the game off in the right frame of mind.

- *Part 2: The Science Of The Nutrition Tower: The Foundations* – This section covers the Foundation Blocks to your Nutrition Tower.

- *Part 3: The Science Of The Nutrition Tower: The Minutia* – Here we delve deeper into refining your Nutrition Tower with the Minutia Blocks.

- *Part 4: Mastering Your Nutrition Strategy And The Smart Shred Diet System* – In this section you're trained to become a strategic player in the nutrition game, and are provided with a "Walkthrough": the Smart Shred Diet System. This system puts together your Nutrition Tower and walks you through a tried and tested Nutrition Strategy to ensure you win at your diet.

- *Part 5: The Loose Ends* – This part covers more specialist strategies, like what to do if your progress stalls, and where you go once you've reached your shredding goal.

- *Part 6: The Round Up* – An emotional debrief.

Key Points

- Some factors of nutrition are far more important to your progress than others.

- Understanding this hierarchy is vital to avoid getting confused by mixed messages about nutrition and fat loss.

- Of all things nutrition, your Calorie intake has the greatest direct impact on your fat loss.

- Next is your protein intake and then your carbohydrate and fat intake.

- Supplements, meal timing, and meal frequency have a much smaller impact on your fat loss than the above, but they can all be important in the right context.

- Calories, protein, fat, and carbs have the greatest direct impact on your results. They're the Foundation Blocks of your Nutrition Tower.

- Other factors can have an indirect impact on your results by modulating those that have a direct effect.

- For example, food quality is extremely important, but quantitatively it won't have a big direct impact on your results. If you eat lots of highly processed foods, you'll feel rubbish, and are unlikely to get your Calorie intake right though.

CHAPTER 3

Why Most People Fail Before They Start: Goals And Expectations

Back when I first hitched onto the nutrition wagon, I was sold on the idea that I could reveal a Herculean physique, with chiseled abs, in a matter of weeks. Given that I was starting from the point of a skinny-fat weedy teen, this was greatly unrealistic. Nevertheless, I did lose fat and began to transform the body I saw in the mirror at, what I now know to be, as an impressive rate.

Despite my reflectively impressive progress, at the time I was disappointed with what I saw, and felt disheartened to have not built a mountain of muscle, shredded a boat load of fat, and reached my goal physique after just a couple of months.

The reason I felt disheartened was that I had no understanding of what a realistic rate of progress was, had naive expectations of what was achievable in the timescale I was working with, and had ultimately set myself an unrealistic goal, which was based purely on the eventual outcome. This is what most people do when they diet; it's why so many fail before they even start and end up throwing in the towel.

So, to ensure you start off on the right foot and get things on point from the go, this chapter is going to cover:

1. What physique transformation you can expect to achieve from applying the information in this book.

2. What the optimum rate of weight loss is to ensure you're shredding fat and not muscle.

3. The simplest and most effective ways to monitor your Smart Shred Diet progress.

4. How long it will take you to get a six pack.

SETTING EXPECTATIONS AND GOALS

Like my former self, many people search for the perfect diet that holds the secret to stacking on muscle, whilst simultaneously stripping body fat.

However, unless you:

- Are a beginner in the gym;

- Have recently lost muscle and are back training again;

- Are particularly overweight;

- Are an assisted trainee (i.e. you take roids)

you can't lose fat whilst building appreciable amounts of muscle, and attempting to do so will just lead to you spinning your wheels and getting nowhere.

So, rather than wasting time wheel spinning, you should:

Focus solely on muscle gain OR fat loss, at any one time

and commit to doing so for at least a couple of months on each occasion (gaining muscle is slower than losing fat; so any massing phase should be longer).

From a quest for cheese grater abs perspective (i.e. shredding/fat loss), the goal is twofold:

- **Lose body fat:** this will reveal the muscle, definition, and physique below.

- **Maintain muscle:** as under most circumstances you can't gain muscle when dieting, so the goal is to maintain as much as possible.

It is this combo that will give your body a strong, toned, and athletic appearance, so, that is what the contents of this book will focus on.*

And with that in mind, we can start to think about appropriate goals and rates of weight loss to aim for. The reason we're working with body weight and not body fat to monitor progress is because it's much simpler and accessible than using reliable body fat estimation tools, and it works as a good proxy for fat loss provided you follow the guidelines of this book.

HOW MUCH WEIGHT SHOULD YOU LOSE PER WEEK TO MAXIMISE MUSCLE RETENTION?

Unlike many others who will give you the bog standard "lose 1lb of weight per week", I like to provide weight loss guidelines based on percentages.

---

*This is assuming you have a sufficient base level of muscle to start with. If you can already see your abs, but haven't got much muscle mass, then it's best to pursue a muscle gaining phase before trying to lose fat, otherwise you'll end up looking skinny, as opposed to muscular, at the end of your diet. There's a video on Bulking Nutrition in the bonus content, so refer to that after reading this book if this relates to you.

Why?

Because it scales, depending on your weight, which is very important given the fact that the more body fat you have on your frame, the faster you can safely drop the pounds without losing muscle.

So, if you're 30% body fat, you could comfortably lose a few pounds of weight per week without compromising muscle. In other words, most of the weight lost would be body fat.

However, if you're 10% body fat, you would sacrifice more muscle if you lost weight at the same rate.

So, a good percentage based goal to aim for is:

0.5–1% weight loss per week.

E.g. If you're 85kg, that would equate to 0.425–0.85kg weight loss per week.

In the initial days/weeks of dieting, you may lose weight at a slightly faster rate than this, which is fine. However, once you start getting deeper into your diet, you should try to stay within this weight loss range for the most part.

HOW TO MONITOR YOUR PROGRESS

To monitor your progress, I recommend a dual approach of **weight recordings** and **progress pictures**.

This is because the scale will give you regular quantitative feedback, which is necessary to assess the effect of your plan, and photos will give you a visual representation of your progress and can act as a massive motivator.

How To Reliably Record Body Weight

I suggest you record your morning weight at least 4 times per week and take a weekly average. It is this average and the trend over time that is important, not the weekly/daily fluctuations as these don't actually reflect changes in body fat.

Have a look at the graph in Figure 7; I've circled two consecutive days, where my weight fluctuated by 2kg.

Unless you're in some Saw-esk film scene where you could lose a limb or two, you can't possibly lose or gain a couple of kgs of body fat over such a short period of time, and in reality, those short term fluctuations reflect changes in:

- Hydration

- Body carb stores

- Poop and wee

- Food in your digestive system

Other factors that may also impact the scale reading include:

- Body fat

- Organs

- The surface your scales are sat on

- The clothes you're wearing

- The scale itself

So, you needn't stress about these short term fluctuations (day to day) and instead, you should keep the bigger picture in mind (weekly and monthly changes). In other words, you should pay more attention to the long term trend, which, in Figure 7, is downwards.

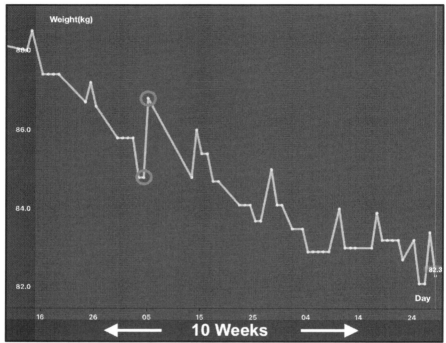

Figure 7.

Because so many factors can bump the scale reading in either direction, when weighing yourself, you need to keep the conditions you record your weight in as consistent as possible.

That means:

- *Clothes:* Wear the same clothes each time. For this reason, I suggest you weigh yourself in your undies only, or in your birthday suit.

- *Time:* Weigh yourself at the same time each day. Ideally it should be done soon after waking up, pre food/drink, and post toilet trip.

- **Scale:** Use the same scale sat on the same surface. Different scales may give slightly different readings and you'll screw up your consistency if one day you place it on your bathroom floor, and the next it's on the carpet. In an ideal world, you should weigh yourself when the scale is sat on a solid surface.

Taking Progress Pictures

I distinctly remember my shock when a disheartened client of mine complained that he wasn't seeing progress in the mirror when to me, his body had completely transformed, and quantitatively his weight had dropped by 6kg in a couple of months. Once I showed him a side by side comparison of his physique when we first started relative to how he looked then, 8 weeks down the line, his opinion completely changed, and he had a revival of motivation as it was so obvious he had made massive progress; day by day he didn't notice changes in the mirror, but his weekly progress pictures told a different story.

This is a great example that shows how pictures are such an effective method of progress tracking, as well as acting as a motivational tool.

Because, in the short term, visual changes aren't as noticeable as weight changes, there's no need to take progress pictures as regularly; so once a week is fine. Like recording your weight, you want to keep things as consistent as possible, and there are a few things to keep in mind when taking your progress pictures:

- **Location:** Ideally take each progress picture in the same place, as the lighting and angle they are taken from will affect the appearance of your physique.

- **Time:** If one week you take your progress picture after a chest and arm training session, you'll look dramatically different relative to one taken another week moments after waking up. This won't give a reliable depiction of your progress; so instead, you should take each picture at the same time of the day, and under the same conditions.

- **Pose:** You need to keep the poses you make for each weekly update the same, otherwise you can't reliably compare pictures. I suggest wearing minimal clothing and tensing. Below are the poses I recommend (full body front, side, and back).

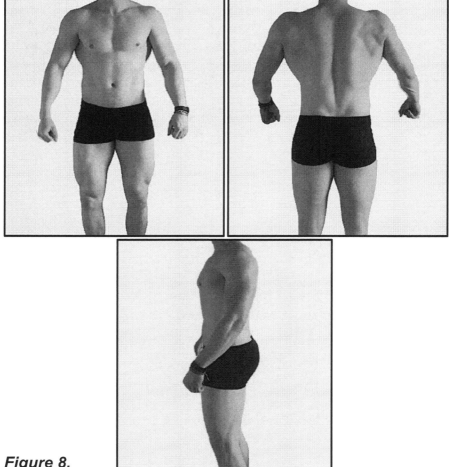

Figure 8.

HOW LONG DOES IT TAKE TO GET ABS?

We live in a society where everyone wants results faster than a kid eats candy.

And this is apparent in the dieting world more so than any other, with book stores being littered with titles promising dramatic results in a matter of days, let alone weeks, months, or even years.

Let me be clear with you though:

If you go into your diet with this quick fix attitude, then you're going to fail somewhere down the line, and any results won't stand the test of time.

So commit to making these dietary changes a lifestyle shift towards a leaner, healthier, and more athletic you.

That's not to say that you'll be dieting for the rest of your life, but following the "Eat Like A Damn Grownup" guidelines in Chapter 9, and having some level of structure to your diet, as covered in Chapter 10, should be carried forward if you want to sustain your results.

The Length Of Your Diet

As for how long your fat loss dieting phase should last, unsurprisingly, it will depend on *[1]* your starting point, and *[2]* how ripped you want to get.

1. Your starting point

If you've got a lot of fat to lose, obviously it's gonna take longer, and vice versa. To quantify where you're starting from, use the chart in Figure 9 to make an estimation of your body fat %. While using the chart to judge your body fat clearly isn't an exact science, it's a quick and effective tool to use for these purposes.

2. How ripped you want to get

Despite us all having different physiologies, for most men, at 10% body fat their abs will start to pop and become defined, as opposed to faint ab groves that appear at higher percentages.

Obviously it's your call on how shredded you want to get, however, for the purposes of standardisation, I feel safe in saying that most guys would love to reach the ab popping threshold of 10%. So, we will use 10% body fat as a standardised goal level of leanness for the rest of this chapter.

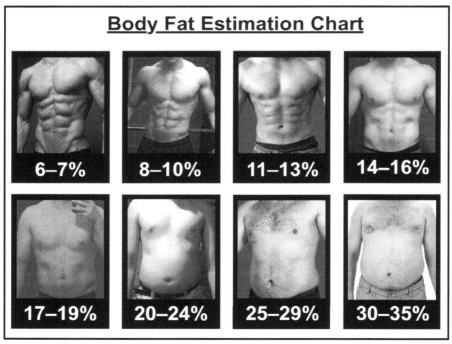

Figure 9.

How long will it will take to get chiselled abs that pop?

With the 10% level of leanness, and your estimated starting body fat percentage in mind, have a look at Table 1 to see how long you can expect to be dieting for.

Starting Body Fat %	Time To Reach 10%
11–13 %	3–6 weeks
14–16 %	8–12 weeks
17–19 %	15–20 weeks
20–24 %	20–30 weeks
25–29 %	32–40 weeks
30–35 %	>40 weeks

Table 1.

Be mindful that these numbers are not set in stone, and it may well take you shorter or longer than the table suggests to get a defined six pack.

This is for a number of reasons:

- The table assumes consistent progress, which in the real world isn't a guarantee.

- Not everyone loses fat at the same rate.

- The rate at which we lose belly fat varies from person to person, as does the rate it's lost from different areas of the body. For example, some people lose fat from their back proportionally faster than their abs. You can't do anything about this, and ultimately it means your abs may pop sooner or later along the dieting line, depending on where you lose fat first.

- You might need to have breaks from your diet. I'll explain this more in Chapter 12, and why purposeful breaks from dieting can actually increase your metabolism, and make your abs more defined in the long run.

So, use the numbers in the table as a means of guidance to give you an idea of the time it will take you to get a six pack.

Key points

- Setting clear and realistic goals is the first step to take.

- Aim to lose 0.5–1% weight per week.

- Record your morning weight at least 4 times per week before eating/drinking, and after going to the toilet. To assess your progress, take an average of these recordings and monitor how your weekly average changes

- Take progress pictures each week in the same location, and under the same conditions.

- Be in this for the long haul, and commit to making long-term lifestyle changes.

- Most guys' abs will start to pop when they're around 10% body fat.

- Use the body fat chart to estimate your body fat percentage, and then refer to the diet duration table to see how long it will take to get ripped abs.

Part 2

THE SCIENCE OF THE NUTRITION TOWER: THE FOUNDATIONS

In this section of the book, you'll learn about the most pivotal factors of your shredding diet, starting with Calories.

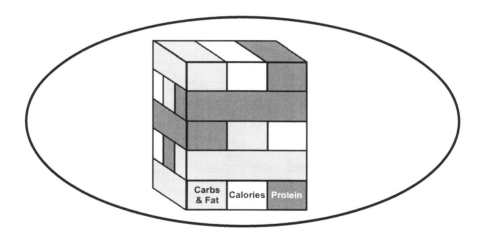

CHAPTER 4

The Poor, Misunderstood Calorie

I feel sorry for Calories.

One minute they're hitting the headlines as the key in the battle against the population's ever growing belly bulge, but the next they're said to be unimportant, insignificant, and secondary to whatever else is being claimed to make us all fat, and sick.

This conflicting information has caused a lot of misunderstanding surrounding the role Calories play in health, fat loss, and six pack endeavours. I've no doubt that it has left you confused at one point or another too.

This chapter will clear up the confusion though, and I want to start off by reminding you of the Jenga concept I introduced earlier, and highlight the position of Calories in the tower: they're slap bang in the middle of the foundation.

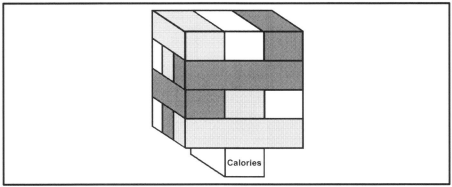

Figure 2.

By the end of this chapter you'll understand exactly why Calories are so fundamental to fat loss, and how to determine you personalised Calorie needs to transform your body.

WHAT ARE CALORIES?

In short:

Calories are simply a unit of measure that we use to express the energy content of food.

So, when you read Calories, think energy.

To put this in a food context, the milk chocolate covered shortbread I had with my tea earlier, racked in at 150 Calories. This means it contained more energy than the 40 Calorie bag of salad I had with lunch. It also tasted approximately 127 times better.

Now, like you fill your car up with fuel to keep the engine running, your body requires energy to fuel all the daily processes it carries out. You know, moving, breathing, organ functioning, and all the other incredible stuff your body does, day to day (seriously, it's insane what your body actually does).

These energy requiring processes can be broken down into 4 categories.

THE 4 COMPONENTS OF METABOLISM

- **Basal metabolic rate (BMR):** The energy you burn at complete rest in a sack-of-potato-like state e.g. lie in bed all day not moving, eating, or drinking.

- ***Thermic effect of feeding (TEF):*** This is the energy burnt after eating/drinking due to the processing of food (i.e. digestion, absorption, fuel storage).

- ***Exercise activity thermogenesis (EAT):*** The energy used during purposeful exercise, like lifting weights.

- ***Non-exercise activity thermogenesis (NEAT):*** This accounts for the energy you burn for all other activities, like walking, fidgeting, and maintaining your posture.

You don't need to know all the intricacies behind the above, but what's important is you're clear that all these processes your body carries out require energy/Calories.

And that this energy doesn't just appear out of thin air, like the excuses when the time comes to train calves; it comes from food, drink, and bodily energy stores.

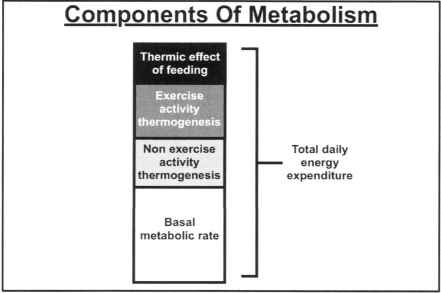

Figure 10.

YOUR BODY IS FUELLED BY THE FOOD AND DRINK YOU CONSUME, AND ITS ENERGY STORES

The Food And Drink You Consume

Cake, chicken, fruit juice, and all that other stuff you shove down your gob contains macronutrients (aka: macros). They are: protein, fat, carbs, and alcohol.

When you digest and process the food/drink you consume, you break chemical bonds in these macronutrients. This breaking of bonds releases energy (Calories) that your body can use to do all the incredible things it does.

Your Bodies Energy Stores

You know that fat you're so desperate to get rid of?

Well, that's one of your body's stores of energy/Calories. When needed, your body breaks down this stored fat of yours for energy. Your body can also store and break down carbohydrates for energy, and can break down muscle and organs to use the protein they're made out of for energy.

So, when your body isn't using the energy from the food/drink you consume to carry out all those bodily processes I mentioned earlier, it draws energy from its own stores:

- body fat,

- stored carbs

- protein in muscles/organs.

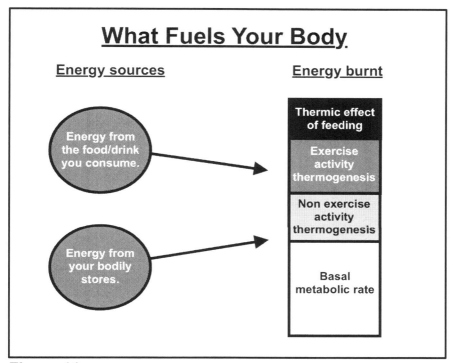

Figure 11.

Over the course of the day, your body jumps between predominantly using its own energy stores as fuel, and the energy that you consume from your diet.

Whether you're burning your own body fat for energy, or the energy you got from your morning croissant at a particular point in time isn't overly important though; it's the balance of your body's use of its own stores (specifically body fat), and your dietary intake over days, weeks, and months that matters.

So, you could wake up, go for a fasted run, and consequently burn a load of fat during the exercise, but in the grand scheme of things, your fat burning workout wouldn't dictate your fat loss.

Likewise, most of the other stuff you've been told about dieting is nonsense.

I'm talking about carbs causing your fat gain, detox shakes being slimming, and coconut oil turning you into a fat-burning machine; you know, the stuff most social media fitness celebs tell you.

Why?

Because no food, drink, or dietary protocol is inherently fattening or slimming; it's the overall Calorie intake that matters.

If there's anything you take away from this book, let it be that last sentence; it will save you a lot of confusion and help you steer clear of all the useless dieting products and protocols that plague the nutrition world.

To expand on this further, I'm going to introduce a phenomenon known as energy (or Calorie) balance; it's the key factor determining your six pack success.

CALORIE BALANCE: THE FAT LOSS SWITCH

As alluded to above, it's the long term balance of your body's energy stores that matters when it comes to fat loss. You see, over the day, you jump between burning and storing your body's energy stores. So you might be burning lots of stored body fat one minute, but then storing a load the next. Again, what's happening at a particular time point isn't all that important; rather, what matters is that over the course of the day/week/month, the sum of the body fat burnt is greater than the amount that is stored. This leads to net fat loss, and you attaining a shredded up, chiselled body. What acts as the switch that drives this net loss of body fat is your Calorie balance, which is the difference between the Calories you consume, and the Calories you burn.

Calorie balance is like a switch that determines whether you have a net gain or loss of body fat.

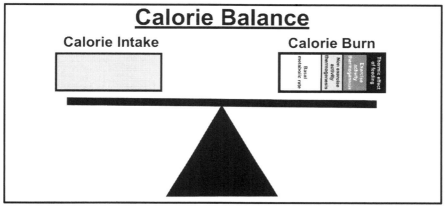

Figure 12.

A Calorie Surplus Causes Net Fat Gain

If you eat more Calories than you burn, you're providing your body with more energy than it needs. Your body isn't dumb, and can't somehow vanish the excess Calories, so it saves them for later by storing them. This results in net storage (gain) of body fat, and weight gain. No matter what you do with your diet, if you are consuming too many Calories (i.e. a surplus), there is no way you can flip the balance to net fat loss as you'll have an excess of Calories ramping up storage.

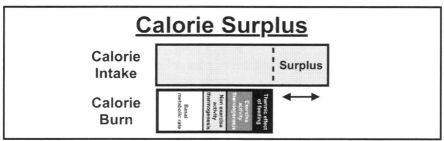

Figure 13.

A Calorie Deficit Causes Net Fat Loss

On the flipside, if you eat fewer Calories than you burn, your body has to sacrifice more of its energy stores to compensate for the lack of Calories coming in from your diet. It also means there are fewer Calories to be stored. Together this combo of greater stored energy usage, and less energy storage leads to net fat loss, and weight loss.

Therefore, a Calorie deficit is what you're aiming to achieve with your fat loss diet, and is why your Calorie intake is the most important factor driving your results.

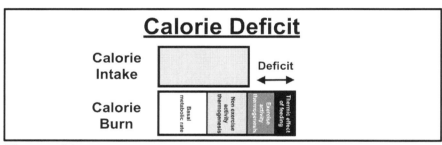

Figure 14.

So, to summarise the above:

- Eat more Calories than your body burns, and you'll put on weight (mostly as fat, unless you lift weights).

- Eat fewer Calories than you burn, and you'll lose weight (mostly as fat, particularly if you lift weights).[*]

That is regardless of how many carbs and doughnuts you eat, whether you eat little and often, and what supplements you take.

---

[*] *Lots of factors can impact what tissue (fat, muscle etc) is lost or gained, but the main point is that you will lose or gain weight based upon your Calorie intake.*

No ifs, buts or questions asked (hence why Calories are head honcho of fat loss).

In fact, you could eat exclusively ice cream, and still lose a shed load of weight and body fat if you got your Calorie intake right. That's not to say that you should, and sure, the specific foods you eat and your meal patterns can have an impact on your results, but their importance is much less so than Calories.

Important Terms To Understand	
Calories	Unit of measure used to express the energy content of food/drink. Much like kgs are to weight, or a mile is to distance.
Calorie Deficit	Calorie intake less than expenditure.
Calorie Surplus	Calorie intake greater than expenditure.
Maintenance Calories	Calorie intake equals expenditure.

Table 2.

So, you MUST consume a deficit of Calories to get a six pack.

And you MUST do this for a prolonged period of time, to see meaningful changes in the mirror (around a month, at the least).

Now, remember earlier, when I mentioned realistic rates of weight loss?

Well, to achieve the 0.5–1% weight loss per week target, you need to consume a deficit of Calories.

The size of the Calorie deficit is important because:

- Too great a Calorie deficit, maintained for a long period of time, will sacrifice muscle, strength, and will just suck in general.

- Too small a deficit will lead to tortoise-like progress.

So, for most people, a good place to start is somewhere in the middle (i.e. a moderate deficit).

Size Of Deficit	% Deficit	Approximate Calorie Deficit	Estimated Weight Loss
Small Deficit	10–15% below maintenance	200–300 Calories below maintenance	0.25kg.per week
Moderate Deficit	20–25% below maintenance	400–600 Calories below maintenance	0.5–1kg per week.
Large Deficit	>25% below maintenance	800–1200 Calories below maintenance	1+ kg per week

Table 3.

From the above table, you can see that a moderate Calorie deficit is roughly 20–25% Calories fewer than your maintenance Calories.

BUT HOW DO YOU WORK OUT HOW MANY CALORIES YOU NEED?

Simple; just follow this two-step process my friend:

Step 1. Use math to get a starting point

There is a boat load of equations you can use to work out your Calorie needs. They all end up giving roughly the same number though; so it's not overly important which one you use. What's important is that you understand they're just a starting point, as they merely provide an ESTIMATION of your Calorie needs.

So pick one, stick with the number it spits out, and it's then up to you to monitor your progress and adjust your Calorie intake after a couple of weeks if needs be.

The equation I recommend

I recommend using the Harris-Benedict (H-B) equation, with an activity factor, to estimate maintenance Calories needs. Essentially, the H-B equation estimates your Basal Metabolic Rate (the number of Calories your body burns in a lay on the bed, sack-of-potato-like state). Then an activity factor is used to account for your daily activities.

So, the H-B equation might give you an estimated BMR of 1500 Calories, and then, if you're moderately active, you would multiply this by 1.55 to give you an estimated daily energy expenditure of 2,325 Calories (which is equivalent to your maintenance Calorie needs).

Go to www.tommycole.co.uk/bookbonuscontent to use the Calorie calculator I recommend for this book.

(If you've got no access to the internet, multiply your body weight in kg by 24 to get a starter Calorie target. This is a very simple, but effective, way to estimate your dieting Calorie needs if you can't use the web link.)

Once you've estimated your maintenance Calories, you need to create a deficit

The above calculator will give you an estimate of your maintenance Calorie needs; so once you've got that, you need to subtract 20–25% of the Calories to create a moderate Calorie deficit.* That's simply a case of multiplying the estimated maintenance Calories by 0.75–0.8.

Using the same example as above, you would end up with 1,860 Calories per day to drop body fat (20% Calorie deficit).

Step 2. Now track your Calorie intake and weight change

After getting your starter Calorie target, you need to monitor your progress, and adjust your Calorie intake if it's not going in the right direction after a couple of weeks of consistent dieting.

For this, you need to download and use a Calorie tracking app for 2 weeks, whilst simultaneously recording your weight as described in Chapter 1. I recommend the MyFitnessPal app to track (visit www.tommycole.co.uk/bookbonuscontent for a tutorial on how to use it).

Based on how your body weight responds to your Calorie intake over the two weeks, you can judge how effective your starter Calorie target is.

---

*Don't do this if you're using the body weight x 24 method.

The Poor, Misunderstood Calorie

- If your weight goes down, you're eating Calorie deficit.

- If your weight goes up over the two weeks or stays the same, your estimation was too high as you're eating a surplus of Calories, or at maintenance, respectively.

(FYI, every 0.45kg – or 1 pound – of weight gained or lost is roughly 3500 Calories. So, if you lost 0.45kg of weight in a week, that would mean you're eating at around about a 500 Calorie deficit each day. Based on this knowledge, you can adjust your Calorie intake accordingly to hit the weight loss rate of 0.5–1% body weight per week.)

As an example, if your weight stays the same, you're eating at maintenance levels, and need to eat 20–25% fewer Calories, to create a moderate Calorie deficit to kick start things.

Chances are your starter Calorie target will be a very good estimate though, and you'll start to see a change in weight right away (within the 2 weeks, that is).

If you feel that you do need to make a change to your Calorie intake:

- Make sure you give it at least 2 weeks of consistent dieting before changing anything; as you can't make a reliable judgement based of a few days or a week.

- I generally suggest doing it in 10% increments. So, if your weight hasn't changed a great deal whilst eating 2000 Calories for a couple of weeks, drop it by 200 Calories, and then reassess after two more weeks. Obviously, there's some trial and error here, and the extent that you change your Calorie intake will depend on how slow or fast your progress is. So, don't see 10% as the magic number.

Key Points

- Calories are a unit of measure for energy.

- Your bodily processes burn energy/Calories throughout the day and night.

- Your body gets the energy to fuel these processes from your diet and bodily energy stores.

- Macronutrients (protein, carbs, fat, alcohol) stored within your body and in the food/drink you consume are where the Calories come from.

- Outside a few special cases, you must burn more Calories than you expend for a prolonged period of time to lose body fat. This is called a Calorie deficit.

- Consuming a 20–25% Calorie deficit will result in roughly 0.5–1% weight loss per week.

- Give it at least 2 weeks of being consistent with your diet before changing anything.

CHAPTER 5

Introduction To Macronutrients And Protein: The Dietary Block Of Strength

In the nutrition world, there's lots of talk about "macros".

And I get that you, being all keen about nutrition, may already know what the deal is with macros. But, to make sure we're both on the same page, over Chapters 6 and 7 I'm going to break down all you need to know about them so you're clued up on exactly how to incorporate them into your programme for the best possible results.

As the name suggests, macronutrients are large nutrients, and they include protein, carbohydrates, fat, and alcohol.

Macros = Macronutrients = Large nutrients

Now, I touched on these macros very briefly, in Chapter 4, when explaining where we get Calories from, so let me recap you on that:

"Cake, chicken, fruit juice, and all that other stuff you shove down your gob contains macronutrients (aka: macros). They are: protein, fat, carbs, and alcohol.

When you digest and process the food/drink you consume, you break chemical bonds in these macronutrients. This breaking of bonds releases energy (Calories) that your body can use to do all the incredible things it does."

So, macronutrients in the food/drink you consume provide you with Calories, as do the macronutrients stored within your body (body fat, glycogen/stored carbs, muscle, organs).

Per gram of each macronutrient, you get:

- Carbohydrate = 4 Calories

- Fat = 9 Calories

- Protein = 4 Calories

- Alcohol = 7 Calories

So, a peanut butter stuffed donut with the following nutritional breakdown:

44g carbohydrate, 25g fat, 9g protein

contains 437 Calories.

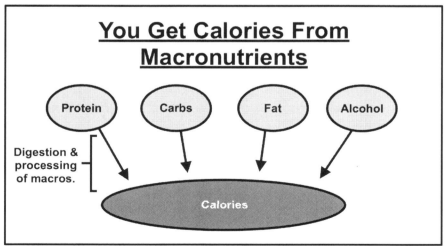

Figure 15.

Now, while all the macros are an energy source, they have distinctive functions, are processed by the body differently, and have varying effects on your body and physique to one another.

So, the rest of this chapter will break down the important stuff you should know about protein – the most important of the macros – and Chapter 6 will then move on to cover fat, and carbs (don't worry; for all my alcohol loving friends, I'll be covering it later on in Chapter 11).

PROTEIN

If Calories are the king of the nutrition world, protein is the prince; it jacks up the muscle building process, it's the most filling of all the macros, and eating it burns more Calories compared to eating fat, carbs, or alcohol.

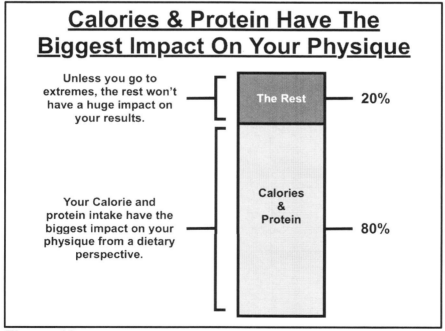

Figure 16.

In fact, a boat load of research tells us that it's the most important macronutrient from a weight and fat loss perspective, with dieters losing more fat, retaining/building more muscle, and feeling more satisfied when consuming moderate to high intakes of the stuff.

This means that after Calories, protein is the most important nutritional factor to get right on your quest for abs.

Now, there are 3 T's you need to consider when it comes to getting your protein intake on point. In order of importance, they are:

1. **Total**

2. **Type**

3. **Timing**

What's that? You're dying to hear more about these three T's? And you want to hear it from me, your favourite of all the blonde, polar bear complexioned nutritionists?

Nawwwww, shucks. Well, I aim to please; so here goes …

1. Total Protein Intake

As with many other nutrition variables, like Calorie intake, the total amount of protein you consume over the course of the day is far more important than any of the other details. So, first and foremost, make sure you pack enough into your diet by eating moderate to high amounts.

To mirror what I told you a second ago, this will lead to greater fat loss, maintenance of muscle mass, and satiety, relative to a low protein intake.

In terms of how much protein to shoot for, I generally suggest:

2g per kg of your target body weight

but anywhere in the region of 1.5–3g per kg of **target body weight** is fine.[*] Because protein helps spare muscle, if you're particularly lean (sub 10% body fat), it's best to aim towards the higher end, whereas if you're not, you've got a little more flexibility.

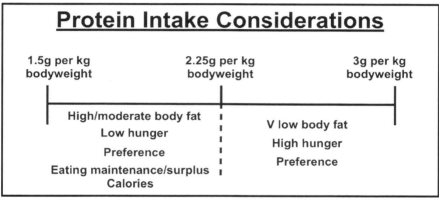

Protein Intake Considerations

1.5g per kg bodyweight	2.25g per kg bodyweight	3g per kg bodyweight
High/moderate body fat Low hunger Preference Eating maintenance/surplus Calories		V low body fat High hunger Preference

Figure 17.

2. Type Of Protein Consumed

While I promised not to get too sciency earlier on, we have to cover some basics of protein biochemistry here (sounds worse than it is). You see, protein is a bit like a big metal chain, in that it's made up of lots of individual links joined up together. The individual links are called amino acids. The specific ones

---

[*]What I mean by your target body weight is your weight in a lean, ab popping state. Don't worry about trying to be really accurate with this; just make a rough estimation of the weight you'd be at with poppin' abs. However, if you're around 15% body fat or lower, just use your current weight, as your target weight won't be hugely different. For the rest of this book, any mention of your body weight in the context of calculating nutrition targets is referring to your target body weight.

that make up a protein, and the way they're joined together determine the quality, and function of the protein.

Of the individual links/amino acids, some are essential and others aren't. When we're talking nutrition, an essential nutrient is one that your body can't make itself, so it must be provided by your diet (remember this, as I'll be bringing it up again later).

So, we need to get some of the amino acids (the essential ones) from our diet more than others (the non-essential ones). Because of this, the quality of a protein is largely dictated by its essential amino acid content:

- **Complete protein**: A protein with all the essential amino acids in the right amounts needed by humans is known as a complete protein and is of high quality. Animal sources of protein are typically complete (e.g. red meat, fish, poultry, eggs, dairy), and there are some complete plant sources too (e.g. quinoa, soybean).

- **Incomplete protein**: A protein with too little of one or more essential amino acid is an incomplete protein and is of lower quality. Plant sources of protein are typically incomplete (e.g. nuts, oats, beans).

Going a little deeper, there are 3 specific amino acids that are more relevant when it comes to building and maintaining muscle. They are leucine, isoleucine, and valine, and together they're known as branched-chain amino acids (BCAAs – no doubt you've heard the term before).

Leucine is particularly important because it ramps up muscle growth maximally when 3g of the stuff is consumed. For most protein sources, you'll get 3g of leucine in a serving size that provides 30–50g of protein.

As an example, 160g of chicken provides around 40g of protein, of which 3g is leucine. Complete protein sources (like chicken) that provide 3g of leucine are great options for your body transformation goals. Table 4 compares other protein sources by their leucine content.

The final factor determining the quality of a protein source is its digestibility. This is what it says on the tin, in that it refers to how easy a protein source is for your body to digest.

Because – unlike animal cells – plant cells have a cell wall, plant sources of protein are typically more difficult to digest. Consequently, we aren't able to make use of as much of the protein contained within plant sources compared to animal sources.

For example, after digestion and absorption, you might attain 80% of the protein available from a serving of kidney beans, whereas you'll get around 95% of the protein contained within a chicken breast. Technically, this means that vegans would likely benefit from eating slightly more protein to compensate for the poorer digestibility. However, from a practical standpoint that may be tricky, and seeing as it isn't a huge deal, I wouldn't get hung up on it if you follow a vegan diet; instead, focus on the vegan guidelines coming your way in a sec.

So, to summarise the above:

- Protein is like a chain, and is made up of lots of individual amino acid links joined together.

- Our bodies' can't make 9 of these amino acids, which are therefore classed as essential amino acids. A protein source containing sufficient amounts of these essential amino acids is a complete protein.

- The amino acid leucine is particularly important for muscle recovery, growth, and retention.

- A high quality protein is one that is *[1]* complete, *[2]* high in leucine, and *[3]* easily digestible.

53

- Animal protein sources meet all of these high quality requirements, whereas plant proteins typically fall short one way or another.

Protein Source	Leucine % Of Total Protein	Approximate Serving Size To Reach 3g Leucine
Whey Protein Isolate	12.00%	30g
Milk Protein Isolate	9.80%	40g
Casein	9.30%	45g
Egg	8.60%	6 eggs
Fish	8.10%	180g
Beef	8.00%	150g
Pork	8.00%	150g
Chicken	7.50%	160g
Wheat	6.80%	15–20 slices of bread[*]

Table 4.

To My Vegan Readership

Now, while this may make it seem as though you should consume only complete sources of protein that are high in leucine to gain/maintain muscle (like meat and dairy), it's context dependent. By that I mean, if you're consuming enough protein in total, then chances are you'll get plenty of the amino

---

[*]*Obviously you're not going to go stuffing your face with 20 slices of bread; that's just there to show how some sources of protein are far suck-ier than others.*

acids required for growth, and you needn't be overly concerned about the sources, complete or not.

I will say that you should try to get your protein from a variety of sources though, particularly if you consume predominantly incomplete proteins, like most vegans. This is because different incomplete proteins can complement one another by providing different amino acids that may be lacking in one source, but not another.

It's a little like the All Blacks compared to a lesser team in rugby. Just as animal proteins are rammed with all the essential amino acids, and are therefore of high quality, the All Blacks are rammed with superstar rugby players and consequently win practically all their matches. Plant sources of protein are like a rugby team with fewer stand out players: individually, they might not be as good, but if the coach selects the right players and their abilities complement one another, they can end up competing against the best.

So, if you eat mostly incomplete proteins (like a vegan would), you need to be a little more aware of the sources you're eating, and aim to get in a greater variety by combining different sources. This ultimately ensures you get in the spectrum of building blocks required for growth.

A simple combination of incomplete proteins that, when eaten together, form a complete protein, is grains in combo with legumes (grains typically lack sufficient amounts of the amino acid lysine, whereas legumes fall short on methionine). If you want to optimise your results while eating a plant based diet, I recommend you combine your incomplete protein sources within meals the majority of the time. This will ensure your muscles are regularly getting all the amino acids they need for recovery and growth. However, if you're not striving to reach the pinnacle of your plant based diet, you needn't combine incomplete proteins at every meal, and will do just fine by getting a variety of sources in over the course of the day. This will make sure your muscles get the amino acids they need for recovery, and the variety of protein sources will also stop your diet from becoming more monotonous than an hour long treadmill slog without a pair of headphones.

3. Timing Of Protein Intake

Whilst the timing and frequency of your protein intake can also be important, as discussed above, what matters the most is your total intake throughout the day. As an example, from a weight/fat loss perspective, a high protein diet is superior to a low protein diet, even if the higher protein intake is consumed in 2 large meals compared to a "little and often" type distribution of 5 meals with the lower protein diet. With that said, to optimise your protein intake, you should divide your total intake between 3–6 meals per day.

I'll be getting into this in more detail later on in the book, but for now, we'll move onto carbs and fat in Chapter 6.

Key Points

- After Calories, protein is the most important nutritional factor to get right when dieting.

- The total amount of protein you consume is the main thing to focus on when it comes to protein intake.

- Roughly 2g of protein per kg of target body weight is a good target to aim for.

- In isolation, animal protein sources are better quality than plant sources.

- Try to consume a diverse array of protein sources.

- Roughly 30–50g worth of protein from a high quality protein source will provide 3g of leucine, and maximise the muscle growth response acutely.

- Ideally, divide your protein intake between 3–6 meals per day.

CHAPTER 6

The Unbiased Truth: Carbohydrate And Fat

By now, you should be pretty clued up on what makes you gain weight/fat; it's not carbs, nor is it fat, but it's a surplus of Calories consumed over a prolonged period of time.

Sure, both carbs and fat provide you with Calories; so they can indirectly make you gain weight if you eat too many, but neither are inherently fattening themselves.

So, neither should be demonised as some sort of dietary devil that's responsible for everything from obesity to the plague, as is often the case. In fact, most people can eat plenty of both whilst dropping the pounds, and thrive on a relatively even balance of the two, which is no surprise considering they both have their own unique roles to play in the body.

FAT

Fat's roles range from cell and hormone production to its use as a fuel source throughout the day and during exercise. This big arse range of roles that fat plays in the body is reflected by the equally big arse range of individual forms of fat, which are split into 3 categories:

- Saturated fat

- Monounsaturated fat

- Polyunsaturated fat

This categorisation comes down to the chemical structure of the different fats, with poly̲unsaturated fats having multiple double bonds in their chemical chain, mono̲unsaturated fats just having one, and saturated fats having none. You don't need to memorise that sciency stuff though; just be sure to remember that there are different forms of fat, and the chemical structure dictates the form.

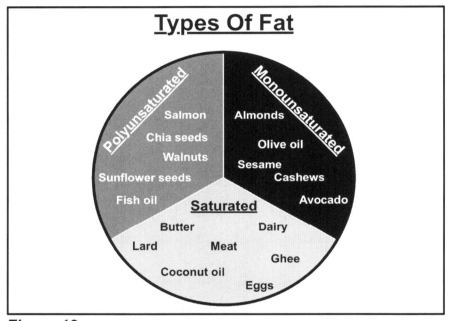

Figure 18.

Whilst you'll hear from various sources that you shouldn't eat a particular category or type of fat (e.g. the whole saturated fat will kill you malarkey), I generally advise to aim for a relatively balanced intake of the three[*]. This is because they all contribute to different aspects of health, and a nutritious and varied diet

---

[*]*Although most sources of fat contain a mix of saturated, monounsaturated, and polyunsaturated fat, I've grouped foods together in Figure 18 to show where you can get the different types of fat from.*

that includes fat sources like meats, eggs, nuts, seeds, dairy, and fish will naturally hit this balanced pattern. So, just keep your intake varied, and don't get too hung up on how much of each type of fat you're packing in.

There Are A Couple Of Exceptions Though

- *Trans fat:* Trans fats are a subcategory of poly-unsaturated fat that are best avoided in their man-made form as the science tells us they're a particularly damaging food molecule that may increase your risk of a load of sucky health conditions. Considering they're pretty much only found in large quantities in highly processed foods, this shouldn't be an issue if you follow the "Eat Like A Grownup" guidelines I'll outline later on in this book.

- *Omega 6 and omega 3 fats:* These are two more subcategories of polyunsaturated fat. Within these categories of polyunsaturated fats are two types of fat that our bodies can't produce and therefore need to be provided by our diets as they're important for lots of bodily functions, including blood flow, immune function, and inflammatory regulation. You needn't worry too much about omega 6 fats, as they're commonly found in lots of foods and if anything, you need to be careful not to over consume them (foods like nuts/seeds, chicken, and vegetable oils are high in omega 6). Omega 3 fats are typically eaten less though, and some of the best dietary sources are oily fish, chia seeds, and walnuts (fish is a better form than veggie sources, which I'll go into later in the supplements section). So, make an effort to get some omega 3 fats into your diet (ideally at least a couple of portions of oily fish each week).

How Much Fat Should You Eat?

In terms of how much fat you should eat, aim for anywhere between 0.5–1.5g per kg of your target body weight. Much below this, and you won't benefit from fat's hunger slashing effects, and you may end up compromising your sex hormone production (e.g. testosterone). On the flipside, if you go too damn high, you'll ramp up Calories pretty sharpish, as fat racks in at 9 Calories per gram, plus you won't leave many Calories left over for carbs, which will likely make your performance in the gym suck balls.

Ultimately, where you fall within this range will depend on a few factors. Namely, your personal preference and activity level. I'll be breaking this down more in a sec after we've covered the sugar glazed doughnutty goodness that is carbohydrates.

KETOGENIC DIETS AND PERFORMANCE

Recently, there's been a lot of hype about ketogenic diets and exercise performance. Ketogenic diets are characterised by very low carbohydrate, but high fat intake, and in most cases, such a diet will compromise exercise performance, making it a poor choice when dieting and trying to maximise muscle retention and performance.

CARBOHYDRATES

Despite what your favourite Instagram fitness bro tells you, carbs aren't the devil, they're not to be feared, and they shouldn't be seen as some sort of enemy to abs.

Like fat, they can be divided into a few different categories, depending on their chemical structure. Typically, they are grouped as:

- *Simple carbohydrates:* these are sugars. Examples of simple carbohydrate sources include: honey, table sugar, syrups, VK Blue, candy, and, well, anything that ever tasted gloriously sweet.

- *Complex carbohydrates:* made up of lots of sugars joined together. They can be 3–10 sugar molecules long (oligosaccharides), or more than 10 (polysaccharides). Oats, potatoes, and the Bible are all examples of complex carbohydrate sources (yeah, you ain't gon' eat a bible, but paper and cardboard are made of complex carbs from wood).

So, carbs are categorised broadly as sugars, or lots of sugar molecules joined together to make a complex carb. Many foods contain a mix of different types of carbs, like a sweet potato that contains both simple and complex carbs, but ultimately, they all end up as sugar once they're dealt with by your body.

You see, when we eat a source of carbs, like a bagel, chocolate bar, or banana, our bodies have to chop up the complex carbs into smaller sugar units, otherwise they're too big to be absorbed.

So, regardless of the source of carbs, they virtually all end up as sugar which then enters our bloodstream. After absorption into the blood, this sugar is then shifted to areas of the body – particularly muscles – where it's either used then and there for energy, or stored as glycogen for use at a later date (glycogen is the stored form of carbs, and despite what fear mongers say, rarely are carbohydrates ever converted to, and stored, as fat). In fact, carbohydrates are such an important energy source our bodies have evolved to make them when we're not getting enough from our diet.

Which leads on nicely to a coupl'a myths about carbs.

Nutrition Myths That Give Carbs A Bad Rep'

Carbs aren't "essential", but that doesn't mean they're unnecessary for optimising your performance

Now, if you've had a few coffees and consequently, your brain is working at double its regular capacity, it may have occurred to you that this ability of your body to make carbs means they're a non-essential nutrient (remember earlier, how I told you a nutrient is technically only essential if your body can't make it itself?). This fact is frequently used against the much-victimised carbohydrate by those promoting low carb diets. However, the reality is that it's just a misinterpretation of what non-essential means, and for those of us carrying out high intensity exercise, dietary carbs are pretty damn important. More on this in a sec.

Carbs raise insulin, but that doesn't mean they make you fat

Another popular argument against carbs – particularly sugar – is that eating them causes a rise in insulin, which in turn, switches off fat burning and ramps up fat storage, subsequently making you a fat-arse. While carbs do increase insulin, which does halt fat burning, to come to the conclusion that this means carbs are inherently fattening ignores the bigger picture of total Calorie intake, and goes against pretty much all the scientific evidence that shows Calories are king. Besides, eating protein also elevates insulin, and last time I checked, no one was calling out a chicken breast and saying it makes you fat.

High GI carbs aren't necessarily bad, nor are low GI carbs universally good

On the topic of insulin, and sugar, you may have heard that simple carbs raise blood sugar quickly and are therefore bad, whereas those that raise it slowly are good (glycaemic index, or GI, relates to how quickly a food raises blood sugar. So high GI carbs raise it quickly, whereas low GI carbs raise it more gradually).

Despite low GI foods generally containing more micronutrients and fibre than high GI foods, there are lots of exceptions and floors with using the GI system to rate carb quality. For example, fructose has a very low GI even though it's a simple sugar, whereas potatoes have a very high GI in spite of them being a complex carb source. Eating other foods with your carbs also alters the blood glucose response to that carb source, making it a pretty dodgy system to use. Besides, looking at individual carb sources in isolation from the rest of your diet is a very narrow-minded way to view things; do you think a bag of skittles is all that bad if the rest of the carbs you eat are fruit and veg? Na, didn't think so.

With that said, as a generalisation, you shouldn't eat that many processed simple carbs, as they're pros at being eaten without filling you up, which puts you at risk of gorging down on too many Calories. So you should try eat mostly complex carbohydrates. Seeing as some very healthy foods, like fruit, contain lots of simple carbs, this clearly isn't a perfect system though. So a good rule of thumb to go by with your carb sources is to:

Eat mostly minimally processed sources of carbohydrate, and one's that contain fibre.

That means mostly complex carbs, and simple carb sources that also contain fibre, like fruit. I'll expand on in this in the Chapter 9, but before all that, we need to cover fibre which, despite being a form of carbohydrate, is handled very differently by your body.

Fibre: A Form Of Carbohydrate Like No Other

While fibre is often thought as separate to carbohydrates, it is technically a form of complex carb, however, we can't digest it like other forms.

What differentiates fibre from the other types of carbs, like starch, is that the bonds joining the sugar molecules together are resistant to human digestion. This inability of your body to break down fibre accounts for its role as a natural bulking agent to foods high in the stuff, which is a big part of fibre's health promoting effects, as it allows food to pass through your digestive system more effectively.

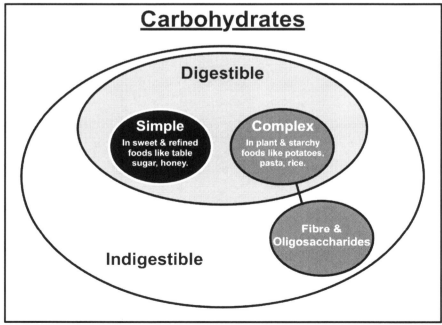

Figure 19.

Other health benefits of fibre include improved blood glucose management, enhanced excretion of potentially toxic substances, and, most relevantly to getting a washboard set of abs, increased satiety, meaning you're less likely to get hungry and pig out if you're eating enough of the stuff.

Now, while your own body cannot break down and digest fibre, as it doesn't have the enzymes to do so, the billions of bacteria residing in your gut can. In other words, fibre is like a big mac for your gut bacteria, and when you eat fruit, veg, and other fibre containing foods, essentially you're feeding the "good" bacteria. As a result of bacterial breakdown of fibre, healthy nutrients are released which your body can absorb and utilise itself. This means that fibre does actually provide you with some Calories (roughly 2–3 per gram) and is another reason why you should be eating sufficient fruit and veg.

A less pleasant, but far more entertaining, by-product of bacterial digestion of fibre is the release of gasses, otherwise known as fart. I like to think I answer the important questions in the nutrition world; so if you've ever wondered why baked beans, Brussel sprouts, and veg in general makes you fart, I'm pleased I've helped you discover the answer. Some oligosaccharides can have a similar effect, which is why many protein bars have warning signs stating that high intakes might cause digestive symptoms.

Summarising the above, fibre is an indigestible carbohydrate that aids digestion, reduces your hunger levels, and can have other healthful effects that may ultimately improve your well-being and lifespan.

As for recommendations, I suggest shooting for roughly:

10–15g of fibre per 1000 Calories, with a minimum intake set at 25g per day.

The reason I suggest setting fibre on a per 1000 Calorie basis is that it scales with the amount of food you eat, which is important considering very high fibre intakes can screw with your digestion and nutrient absorption.

With all that said, provided you actually eat like a grownup and get a variety of fruit, veg, and whole grains in, you needn't worry about paying too much attention to the exact amount of fibre you eat, as you'll meet these targets by default.

And on that note, we'll move onto:

SETTING FAT AND CARB TARGETS

As I mentioned earlier, your fat intake depends primarily on your preference and activity level, which by default, means your carb intake also depends on these factors, as carbs and fat make up the remaining Calories after you've determined your protein intake.

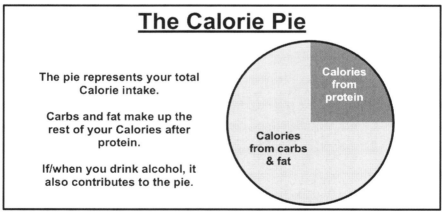

Figure 20.

Preference

Preference is pretty self-explanatory, and you're the best judge of your likes/dislikes, and how easily you'll be able to stick to different intakes of carbs and fat.

Activity level

When it comes to your activity level and performance, we need to look at the intensity of the exercise you're doing.

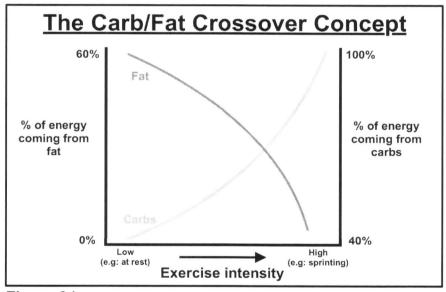

Figure 21.

You see, at high intensities, you require fast acting energy sources to fuel the work you do. Because it takes a long time to yield energy/Calories from fat relative to carbohydrates, they're out of the picture when exercising at a high intensity, and therefore, most of the energy you burn comes from carbs.

So, when doing high intensity exercise, like lifting heavy weights, and sprinting, the majority of the energy you burn is from carbs. However, at lower intensities when you don't require energy at such a rapid rate, it makes sense for your body to shift its energy yield to fat, as it has much higher stores of the stuff. So, at rest, and when doing low intensity exercise like light jogging, you'll use mostly fat as fuel. As always, in the nutrition world, there are ifs and buts here, however, this carb–fat crossover concept is generally how things work.

BURNING FAT ISN'T THE SAME AS LOSING FAT

While I didn't intend this book to include much on cardio (because, well, screw cardio), this is a good time to point out that whilst you do burn a greater proportion of fat during low intensity exercise, that doesn't mean low intensity cardio makes you lose fat. The same goes for other diet and exercise factors that cause you to burn more fat acutely, like fasted cardio.

Yeah, I know, that doesn't seem to make a lot of sense. So let me quickly explain.

How come burning more fat during exercise doesn't necessarily lead to fat loss?

I like analogies, so I'm going to use one here. I want you to think of fat loss like your financial status whereby, you won't instantly become broke after going out for an expensive dinner (unless you're an idiot, or you end up getting drunk and hitting the casino). Sure, it may put a momentary hole in your pocket, but your overall financial status is dictated by the money going in and out of your account over weeks, months, and years; not acute moments throughout the day (again, unless you're an idiot).

Fat loss is like this: it's the result of the long term balance of fat storage and loss, which is primarily dictated by the number of Calories you eat, relative to how many you burn. So, just because you burn more fat doing low intensity Cardio, it doesn't mean it will cause a net loss of fat over the day/week/month. By no means is that to say it's a bad method of cardio, it's just an important point I wanted to make. Now, back to carb and fat recommendations.

So, taking this all into account, the greater the volume of high intensity exercise you do, the more you will need to skew the balance of your fat–carb intake towards carbs, in order to fuel performance, and muscle, and strength gains/maintenance. Below are a few more of the considerations to make with your fat–carb balance.

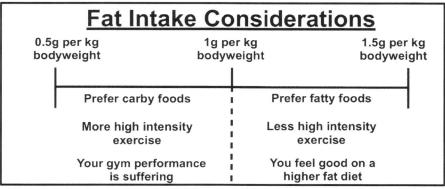

Figure 22.

Once you've decided whether to go low or high on the carb–fat front, simply choose a fat target that reflects this on the range I mentioned above (0.5–1.5g per kg target body weight).

If you're unsure, go for 1g of fat per kg of target body weight.

You then need to take the remaining Calories and convert them to grams of carbs. To do this, divide the Calories left over by 4.

71

As an example, let's take a hypothetical 80kg bro I've named Ricky P, who has Calculated he needs 2000 Calories per day to lose weight/fat:

- If he goes for a standard protein intake of 2g/kg body weight, that gives a protein target of 160g per day.

- He does a moderate amount of high intensity exercise, and likes both carby and fatty foods equally; so has gone for 1g of fat/kg body weight, giving 80g of fat per day.

- Now he needs to work out how many Calories that leaves left for carbs. Because protein is 4 Calories per gram, and fat is 9 Calories per gram, that means multiplying his protein target by 4, and his fat target by 9, then subtracting the sum of these two from his total Calorie target. Like this:

$$(160 \times 4) + (80 \times 9) = 1360$$
$$2000 - 1360 = 640$$

- So, 640 Calories left over for carbs. Because carbs are 4 Calorie per gram, he divides 640 by 4 to give 160g of carbs as his daily target.

Along with the fibre guideline of 10–15g per 1000 Calories (with minimum of 25g per day), these steps give Ricky P the following daily nutrition targets:

2000 Calories
160g protein
80g fat
160g carbs
25–30g fibre

Simple as that.

Provided Ricky P consistently hit those targets, with some degree of precision, he would strip down the body fat and uncover his abs, regardless of any other nutritional factors, such as the time he eats his meals, the types of foods he eats, and the amount of sugar in his diet.

I'll be breaking down the various methods you can use to hit these targets in Chapter 10, but next up is Part 3, where we'll be covering the blocks that refine your Nutrition Tower.

Key Points

- Carbs and fat make up the rest of your Calorie intake after protein (excluding alcohol).

- Neither are inherently fattening or unhealthy.

- Carbs aren't essential in the technical sense of the word, but they're a very important fuel source for high intensity exercise.

- Consider your personal preference and activity level when determining your carb, and fat intake.

- Set your fat intake to reflect your preference (high/low fat/carbs).

- Consume 0.5–1.5 g of fat per kg of target body weight and the rest of you Calories as carbs. 1 g of fat per kg target body weight is what I recommend if you're unsure.

- Aim for a minimum of 25g of fibre per day.

PART 3

THE SCIENCE OF THE NUTRITION TOWER: THE MINUTIA

This section covers nutritional factors that will refine your Nutrition Tower. These blocks don't have a huge impact on your progress relative to the 3 Foundation Blocks, but in the right context, the minutia can be important. To recap, the Minutia Blocks I'm referring to are your meal timing, meal frequency, and supplements.

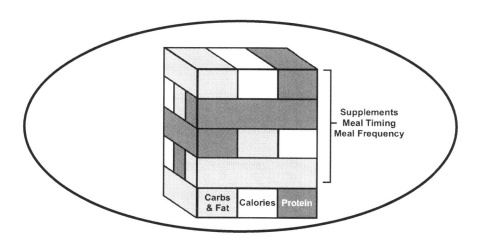

CHAPTER 7

When To Major In The Minor: Meal Timing And Frequency

At this stage, you know more than enough about nutrition to transform your body. In fact, you know more than 96.5641% of anyone who ever journeyed on a quest for cheese grater abs. Ok, that's not a legit stat; but I mean it when I say that most people don't know this stuff.

Seriously, you'd see incredible results if the recommendations prior to this section are all you take forward into Part 4 of the book, where you'll go through a process of setting up a personalised diet.

However, in this next part of "The Science Of The Nutrition Tower", you're going to learn how to refine your Nutrition Tower by careful implementation of the Minutia Blocks.

I refer to these factors as the Minutia Blocks simply to jam home the point that they are far from central to your body transformation results, and because many dieters balls up by prioritising them from the off, in preference over the Foundation Blocks. In other words, they major in the minor, getting distracted by inferior nutrition variables.

This doesn't make the Minutia Blocks unimportant though, and there certainly is a time and a place to knuckle down on these blocks of your Nutrition Tower, which you'll be fully clued up on by the end of the next couple of chapters.

The Minutia Blocks of your Nutrition Tower are grouped into 3 categories:

- **Meal frequency:** e.g. eating little and often to boost metabolism.

- **Meal timing:** e.g. having a shake immediately post workout.

- **Supplement**s: e.g. fat burning supplements.

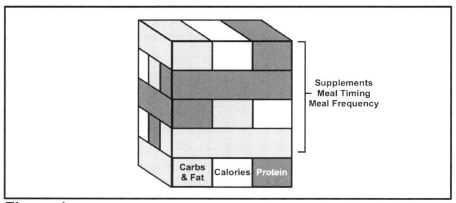

Figure 1.

To expand upon the Jenga analogy earlier, this is how they fall into the nutrition hierarchy for fat loss:

Calories → Protein → Carbs and fat → Meal frequency and meal timing → Supplements

So, your Calorie intake is more important than the amount of protein you eat, which is more important than your carbohydrate and fat intake, which is more important than meal timing and frequency, which …

Well, yeah; you get the point.

Having already covered the foundational nutrition variables, we will now continue in order of importance, starting with meal frequency and timing, and then, move on to supplements in Chapter 8, which is synonymous to the cherry that tops your nutritional cake.

MEAL FREQUENCY

The most prevalent belief here is that eating little and often spikes metabolism, and consequently leads to fat loss, and you becoming a ripped-arse cover model. While there is some legitimate science that underpins this idea, in reality, things don't pan out like the "little and often" proponents will have you believe.

Let me explain …

Should You Eat Little And Often?

If you track back to what we covered earlier about metabolism, you might remember that some of the energy you burn day to day (around 5–10%) is due to you digesting/processing food and drink (the thermic effect of feeding). So when you eat, your metabolism does go up. This is the science that drives the "eat little and often" belief, as it would seem that spiking your metabolism more frequently, by eating lots of meals, would lead to more Calories burnt overall and therefore, more weight/fat loss.

Thing is, if you eat the same total amount of food over the course of the day, the effect that your feeding frequency has on your metabolism is negligible. This makes a lot of sense if you think about it intuitively. To help explain why your meal frequency isn't a big deal when it comes to your waistline, I want you to take yourself back to the last time you felt full. I'm talking about the type of fullness you get post-Christmas dinner. You know, yoga ball food baby full. Pretty uncomfortable, wasn't it?

Imagine how much time and effort it took for that food baby to be broken down, processed, and absorbed by your body. It would have required a lot of energy, that's for sure. You might have been so full that you even had to go out for a stroll to help your belly with the digestion.

Now, compare that to the effort it would take to quickly scoff down and process a small bowl of coco pops. In comparison, the effort and energy required from your body to process this small meal would be much less.

The point I'm getting at here is that the increase in metabolism as a result of a meal is proportional to its size, with larger meals having a greater boosting effect than smaller ones.

So, while eating little and often will increase your metabolism more frequently, each boost will be smaller than if you were to go for fewer but larger meals.

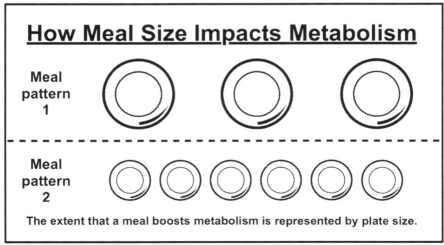

Figure 23.

For example, let's say that one day you decide to eat lots of little meals because Guy – your hench mate down at the local gym – told you it would keep your metabolic fire roaring. Each meal would increase your metabolic rate slightly, adding up to maybe 200 Calories burnt from the thermic effect of feeding over the course of the day, if you were to eat 2000 Calories in total.

If you were then to eat fewer, but larger meals the next day, each one would increase your metabolic rate to a greater degree than the individual meals the previous day. Provided you were to eat the same total amount of food over the course of the day (2000 Calories worth), the larger meal size would compensate for the lower meal frequency, adding up to the same 200 Calorie boost in metabolism as the previous day's meal pattern.

So, in a nutshell, despite being jacked, tan, and strong as a silverback, your mate Guy was wrong, as it is the total amount of food over the course of the day that determines how much your metabolism increases from eating, not the frequency of your meals. Besides, the thermic effect of food only adds up to around 5–10% of your overall daily Calorie burn, and you can't do a great deal to increase it other than eat more food in general; so, you shouldn't get hung up on any so-called metabolism boosting strategy, diet, or food.

To Maximise Your Results, You Should Space Your Protein Out

Now, while you needn't be overly concerned about your meal frequency, particularly from a metabolism boosting perspective, there is a case for spreading your protein intake out over 3–6 meals per day. Don't get me wrong, this won't make or break your results, like Guy would probably tell you, but it will help you maximise them if that's what you're going for.

You see, when you eat protein, you stimulate the muscle growing process. The stimulatory effect of a protein feed on muscle is maximised at a dose of 30–50g (which is a standard chicken breast or a scoop of protein), and any extra protein won't have a great deal of added benefit acutely. This elevation, in muscle growth, as a result of an "optimal" dose of protein, then lasts for around 3–4 hours. So, theoretically, if you were to eat 3–6 meals containing at least 30–50g of protein, you would spike muscle growth a number of times throughout the day as opposed to just once or twice, like a lower, less optimal, frequency would do. More than 6 meals per day would also be a sub-optimal feeding strategy, as it would reduce the dose of protein per meal to a sub-optimal amount, and the time between meals would be too short to maximise the growth response your muscles make to protein.

While stimulating muscle growth a number of times per day by eating protein won't necessarily lead to net muscle growth during your diet (similarly to how acute changes in fat burning don't dictate overall fat loss), distributing your protein over 3–6 meals will likely help you retain muscle to a degree.

So, if you want to maximise your results, space your protein intake out relatively evenly, between 3–6 meals per day. Again, it won't be the factor that determines if you get ripped, Thor-esk abs, or beach ready, but it will likely have a small effect.

MEAL TIMING

Despite what Guy – your well-meaning, but ill-informed friend – tells you, you don't have to chug a shake the second you drop the dumbbells on your last set of curls, you won't necessarily get fat if you eat carbs after 8pm, and eating breakfast, sure as hell, isn't required to kick start your metabolism.

In other words, like meal frequency, the time you eat isn't a big deal from a physique perspective.

Nevertheless, in the right context, meal timing can be somewhat important.

So, the three main meal timing topics I'm going to cover in this section are:

- The post workout anabolic window and nutrition around training.

- Will eating at specific times make you fat?

- The breakfast myth.

We'll start with the anabolic window, as it ties in with what's just been covered on meal frequency.

Is There A Post Workout Anabolic Window?

The 30 minutes, or so, post workout are often believed to be vital to your body transformation success, in that it's a time when your muscles are primed for growth and are sat waiting for an anabolic influx of nutrients. This has led to many lifters religiously downing a shake containing a mix of protein and simple carbs; the two nutrients said to maximize growth in the post workout window.

Without meaning to sound like a scratched Justin Bieber CD (i.e. the WORST kind of broken record), by now, it should be clear to you that it is your total daily intake of nutrients that has the greatest impact on your results, and the time of a shake shouldn't be number one on your nutrition priorities list.

In the right context, a post workout protein or a protein/carb feed is beneficial though, and may help maintain your gains and performance when dieting.

Protein post workout

As mentioned earlier, after you eat protein, muscle growth is elevated for a few hours before dropping back down to baseline levels. This means that the benefit of protein post workout depends on when your last feed of the stuff was.

For example, if you ate a meal containing 30–50g of quality protein an hour or so before training, you'll still have plenty circulating in your system for your muscles to suck up for growth. So, in this context, you shouldn't fuss about having another protein feed immediately post workout. However, if you went into a training session without consuming protein in the 3–4 hours prior, getting some in shortly after your session (within an hour or so) will help maximise your progress by re-spiking growth.

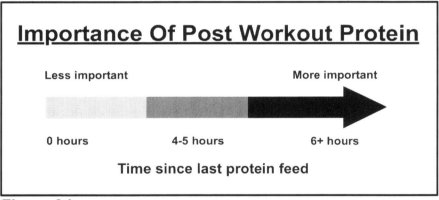

Figure 24.

Carbs post workout

Some claim that carbs added to protein increase the muscle growing response to a meal, as it increases insulin release (a hormone with anabolic and anti-catabolic effects). However, this is not the case if your protein dose is sufficient (30–50g or more), as consuming protein (particularly a fast digesting protein like a whey shake) elevates insulin levels too, and will do so enough to maximise insulin's effects on muscle growth. So, don't think that adding carbs to your protein shake will further increase your gains or maintenance of muscle/strength during a diet.

Adding carbs might benefit your performance if you're training the same muscle group hard twice in one day though. This is because, post gym sesh, when you've got your sweat on, squatted the equivalent of an oak tree, or curled enough to leave you with Michelin Man like guns, you will have depleted your muscles' stores of carbohydrate (i.e. glycogen; the energy storage form of carbs) to some degree. This leaves your muscles like a sponge to carbs for a short period of time post lifting, and in this time they will quickly soak up the carbs you consume to restore glycogen levels.

This short period, where your muscles rapidly soak up carbs, is called Phase 1 of glycogen resynthesis, and lasts 30–60 minutes post workout.

If you're only training once in a day, then making use of this sponge like muscle sensitivity to carbs isn't important, as the 24 hours, or so, between sessions is more than enough time to ramp your bodies carb stores/glycogen back up using Phase 2 (the slower phase); that is provided you eat enough carbs in total.

If you are training the same muscle group twice in a day though (e.g. having a high volume leg session in the morning and then going to rugby training later on), it's beneficial to make use of Phase 1 by eating around 1–1.5g/kg body weight of carbs within an hour after your first session, so you have plenty of energy stored for your second.

E.g. in a food context, that might be 100g of oats made with milk, and topped with a banana for a 70–80kg male. Obviously, that is provided it fits within your daily nutrient requirements.

Will Eating At Specific Times Make You Fat?

The primary concept that pops to mind here is that eating carbs after 8pm makes you fat because you don't burn them off when you're asleep. Thing is, you don't suddenly stop burning Calories when you're asleep because your organs are still functioning. Well, unless you're dead that is.

So simply put, the answer is no; eating at certain times won't make you fat.

And again, without meaning to sound like a scratched-up Justin Bieber record, regardless of whether you eat a big bag of popcorn seconds before you fall asleep or not, it's your total Calorie intake relative to your expenditure, over the day/week/month/year, that determines your waistline. So, don't stress about eating carbs or whatever else after 8pm, provided your total intake is on point.

The Breakfast Myth

Like eating late on in the evening won't make you fat, eating breakfast won't rev up your metabolism and make you look like Greek god either; remember, your metabolism doesn't suddenly stop overnight; so if it needed kick starting in the morning like so many claim, it would mean you're dead.

As previously discussed, if you're looking to maximise your results, spacing your protein out over the course of the day is advisable though, which means getting some in during the morning is sensible. However, it is by no means necessary, particularly if it doesn't fit your preferences and lifestyle.

Because a lot of people train in the morning, I will add that having a breakfast containing 30–50g of quality protein soon after a morning session is advisable, seeing as you won't have eaten anything overnight and consequently gone without protein for a long time. That might simply be a protein shake, some eggs on toast, or some Greek yogurt with berries, for example. Either that, or get in a quick protein shake or something similar just before your session (this is one of the only occasions where I would consider advising a BCAA supplement. More on this in a minute though). The reason for this recommendation comes back to what I said about post workout protein above, and its importance in relation to when your last feed was.

INTERMITTENT FASTING IS A STRATEGY TO IMPROVE ADHERENCE: NOT SOME MIRACLE DIET

Recently, in the nutrition world, there has been a lot of praise for intermittent fasting, which for those without the foggiest of what I'm on about, is a meal timing strategy whereby you restrict when you eat to a certain time window. So you might fast from 8pm until 12pm the next day, for example. This fasting pattern would give you an 8-hour window to eat your day's food.

Going by the way some people talk of intermittent fasting, you might think it's some form of miracle diet that will make you lose weight faster, whilst being able to eat whatever you want. This simply isn't the case though, and from a weight/fat loss perspective, it's merely a tool that may ultimately help you eat fewer Calories than you burn.

It can help you achieve this by:

- ***Improving your hunger awareness:*** Many of us go without ever feeling true belly rumbling hunger because we reach for a chocolate bar or whatever else the second hunger strikes, and have become accustomed to eating regularly purely out of habit. When you get accustomed to fasting, you learn to appreciate hunger, you recognise that it's no big deal, and that you can comfortably go about your day without needing to eat every couple of hours.

- ***Suiting your lifestyle and preferences:*** This makes you more likely to stick out your diet long term.

- ***Making you feel full:*** If you space your meals out throughout the day, you may feel you're never fully satiated. If, however, you restrict your meals to an 8 hour or so time window, you may be much more satisfied after each meal.

- ***Enabling you to eat with more freedom:*** This is because you'll have a big chunk of Calories to play with in your eating window. Even if you don't fast every day, intermittent fasting is a good strategy to implement for social occasions, like on days where you're eating out with friends and when in other similar situations.

- ***Providing an extra level of structure to your diet:*** This allows you to control your Calorie intake better.

I myself used an intermittent fasting structure on my recent diet by skipping breakfast and eating my first meal at 2pm. Because I don't get very hungry in the morning, it worked well for me, and made my diet almost effortless as I had lots of Calories for later in the day. In other words, it fit my lifestyle and preferences. This (personal preference) is the primary factor you should take into account when deciding whether to give intermittent fasting a go or not. The same goes for any other meal timing/frequency strategy, as going with one that suits you and your lifestyle will help you eat a deficit of Calories, and stick out your diet long term.

Key Points

- The hierarchy of nutrition for fat loss is: Calories → Protein → Carbs and fat → Meal frequency and meal timing → Supplements.

- To maximise your results, space your daily protein intake out relatively evenly between 3–6 meals per day.

- If you don't consume protein within 3–4+ hours prior to training, it's a good idea to get 30–50g in soon after your session.

- Carbohydrates post training are most important if you train the same muscles twice in a day.

- The time you consume your Calories has little, if any, direct impact on your fat loss and won't affect your metabolic rate to any meaningful degree.

CHAPTER 8

The Cherry That Tops Your Nutritional Cake: Supplements

Back in my early days of lifting, I remember thinking whey protein was steroid-like in its effects on muscle growth, BCAAs were the secret to sleeve-hugging biceps, and that taking creatine was verging on substance abuse. In fact, the supplement companies had me believe all kinds of nonsense with their anabolic this and that labelled products; I guess Guy must have worked for them.

Now I understand that it's simply not the case, and the reality is that any supplement you can legally buy in a store or online is, at best, a cherry on top of your nutritional cake.

So, first and foremost, you should focus on all the nutrition variables discussed in the chapters prior to this one, and then, if you've got some spare cash going, you might want to add in some supplements that actually have robust scientific evidence to support their use (unlike the vast majority of those on the market).

Obviously, if you're deficient in one nutrient or another, taking a supplement to correct that will be beneficial, regardless of your diet. However, I'm coming from the angle that you're consuming a nutritious diet that meets your basic needs. In that context, only a select few supplements will provide you with any benefit, which I discuss below.

CREATINE MONOHYDRATE

Effects and use: The molecule creatine helps produce energy during high-intensity exercise lasting between 0–6 seconds. So, think heavy-arse lifting, and explosive exercise like sprinting. It is the most well-researched supplement for weight training, and the overwhelming majority of studies show that its long-term use improves strength and muscle size. As with all supplements, there is individual variation in responsiveness, and when it comes to creatine, those most likely to benefit the most are vegetarians/vegans, as creatine is naturally found in meat.

How to take: While there are lots of different forms of creatine on the market, creatine monohydrate is the most well researched, and you shouldn't bother with any other forms, regardless of the claims on the tub. As for dose, if you need to improve your performance quickly for one reason or another (e.g. within a week or 2), take a loading dose of 0.3g per kg of body weight per day for 5 days, and then, transition onto a maintenance dose of 5g per day. This will ramp up your muscle stores of creatine quickly. Most people have no need to do this though, and should simply take 5g per day from the off. The time you take it doesn't matter, and what's important is your consistent daily supplementation, as it's all about building up and maintaining elevated muscle creatine stores.

Additional information: Because creatine is shuttled into muscles along with water, when you initially start taking it, you may gain some weight, or not lose it as quickly if you're dieting. This is merely water being retained within your muscles and nothing to do with body fat; so it's nothing to worry about. In fact, it will make your muscles look a little fuller.

CAFFEINE

Effects and use: Like creatine, caffeine is a highly studied performance supplement. Its main use is as a stimulant, but caffeine also increases metabolism in the short term. Whilst this acute boost in metabolism might seem great, I want to point out that this effect of caffeine is nothing to call home about, and doesn't translate into meaningful physique changes. So, I want you to just view it as a tool you can use pre-workout, to reduce fatigue and give you a boost when needed. The kick-up-the-arse-like stimulatory effects of caffeine are thanks to it blocking receptors in the brain responsible for relaxation.

How to take: 3–6 mg per kg of body weight taken 30–60 minutes pre-workout is the dose supported by science, however, there is a great deal of individual variation in response to caffeine intake. So you need to consider your personal tolerance and how it affects you individually. To put this into real life context, a regular/medium Americano you might buy from a cafe, like Starbucks or Costa, racks in at roughly 200–300 mg of caffeine, which would hit the lower end of the recommendation for most men.

Additional information: It should come as no surprise that I don't advise you to consume caffeine late on in the day, as it has the potential to screw with your sleep and recovery if you do. You see, caffeine has a half-life of around 5–6 hours, meaning that it takes 5–6 hours for half of what you consume to get out of your system. So, as an example, if you have a coffee or caffeine-containing pre-workout supplement just before an 8pm training sesh, you'll still have plenty flowing through your system when you hit the sack later on (assuming you're not some nocturnal night owl). It's also worth noting that some people can suffer some sucky side effects of caffeine, particularly at high doses. These include anxiety, headaches, and restlessness, but you probably know if you suffer from these already.

BETA ALANINE

Effects and use: You know that burning sensation you get during a high rep set of curls, leg extensions, or whatever other exercise you're doing? Well, that's thanks to metabolites, like hydrogen ions, that build up in your muscles as a by-product of high intensity energy production. When hydrogen ions build up in a muscle, the muscle's acidity increases too, which leads to the burn you feel, and a drop in your performance. Where beta alanine comes into all this is its role as a precursor to a molecule called carnosine, which is one of the muscles' main acid buffers. So, when you take beta alanine, you increase levels of carnosine, which gives you a greater ability to combat the acid built up during high intensity exercise. Ultimately, this may help you maintain your strength and ability to squeeze out a couple more reps during high rep sets lasting around 60 seconds, or throughout a high-volume training session.

How to take: Because the benefits of beta alanine supplementation come with the coinciding increase in muscle carnosine stores, you need to take it consistently, over a prolonged period of time, to build and maintain carnosine levels. 3–4g taken consistently, every day, will do this over time. Like creatine, the time you take beta alanine doesn't matter, and you can take the 3–4g dose all at once. Because it can cause a tingly sensation, some people like to divide their daily dose into 2, as the tingles are dose dependent.

Additional information: As mentioned above, beta alanine can make your skin tingle. As of yet, there is no evidence to suggest this is a bad thing other than it being uncomfortable for some people, and there have been no other observed side effects of beta alanine supplementation at a 3–4g per day dose.

CITRULLINE MALATE

Effects and use: This is a combo of citrulline and malate, which when combined together, may have synergistic effects on performance. Despite working via different mechanisms, citrulline malate is somewhat similar to beta alanine, in that it may boost performance by delaying the build-up of metabolites during high volume sets and sessions. This means it may ultimately enable you to get in a few more reps during high volume training sessions, which will improve your physique over time.

How to take: 8g taken 60 minutes pre-workout has been shown to improve high volume weight training performance. In this instance, the timing counts; take it 30–60 minutes pre-workout.

Additional information: Citrulline malate is a relatively new supplement on the scene, however, the existing research is promising, hence it's inclusion here.

PROTEIN POWDER

Effects and use: A protein supplement is, by no means, necessary, and should merely be seen as a cheap and easy way to help meet your total protein requirements. As for the form of protein you go for, dairy sources are generally better than plant sources. There is no need to stress over fast digesting this, or sustained release that. It really makes very little difference, and for most, a bog-standard whey protein concentrate is the most cost-effective option. So, ignore the marketing claims for the most part, and instead look out for the amount of protein you're getting per 100 Calories. If it's 18g, or more, per 100 Calories (or roughly 80+g per 100g of powder), then it's most likely a decent option to go for.

How to take: Just take it as and when to help meet your protein needs. Don't overdo the stuff though, as it won't fill you up as much as whole food sources of protein.

Additional information: If you're a vegan and you don't want to go for a whey supplement, pea protein is a relatively good alternative, as are blends of pea, hemp, and rice (remember, legume and grain sources of protein complement each other to make a complete protein).

Other supplements that aren't typically marketed for athletic performance or body composition

The above covers almost all the supplements that are worth your hard-earned cash, particularly from a performance and body composition perspective. However, some nutrients are commonly under consumed, so I wanted to mention them quickly, here too.

MULTIVITAMIN/MINERAL

Effects and use: While you should be all set from a vitamin and mineral standpoint if you eat a variety of whole foods, as outlined in Chapter 9, a multivitamin will add an extra level of security against nutrient deficiencies and illness. This is more relevant when you're dieting, as you'll most likely be eating less in general, and will consequently be getting fewer nutrients in.

How to take: There's no need to go for a mega-dosed multi, particularly if you're eating a nutritious diet in the first place; so a regular one a day multivitamin will do the job.

Additional Information: Nada.

ESSENTIAL FATTY ACIDS/FISH OIL

Effects and use: Remember earlier, when I explained how it's important to get some omega 3 fats in your diet and that fish/seafood sources are generally better? Well, this is because seafood provides forms of omega 3 fats called eicosapentaenoic acid (EPA) and docosahexaenoic acid (DHA), which are the forms that give rise to most of the health-promoting benefits of omega 3 fats. While still being solid choices, vegetarian sources provide us with an omega 3 fat called alpha-linolenic acid (ALA), which has to be converted to EPA and DHA before we benefit most from its consumption. This conversion of ALA is very inefficient, so it's best to get some omega 3s from seafood if possible. If, like me, you're not all that big a fan of seafood and eat very little, then supplementing with a fish oil may be beneficial and, among other potential benefits, could help with joint recovery and circulation.

How to take: If you don't eat much oily fish (<2x per week), 1–2g of fish oil with an EPA to DHA ratio of 2:1 has been recommended for athletes.

Additional information: Polyunsaturated fats, like those found in fish oil, are particularly fragile and susceptible to damage from light and heat. So, make sure that you keep any fish oil supplement in the fridge, out of light, and ideally buy one that's kept in an opaque tub.

VITAMIN D

Effects and use: Many people, particularly those with dark skin in countries without much sun, have low levels of vitamin D. Seeing as vitamin D is damn important for a bazillion different bodily functions, which include maintaining bone health, muscle function, and testosterone levels, it's well worth having your levels checked, and potentially considering a supplement if you're rarely exposed to sun.

How to take: The appropriate dose depends on your current levels and sun exposure; so it's best to have a test done first. 400–2,000 IU/day of vitamin D3 is sufficient for most who choose to supplement.

Additional information: Along with vitamins A, E, and K, vitamin D is classed as a fat soluble vitamin. This means that – unlike the water soluble vitamins – it can be stored in your body, and if you take very high quantities of it, your stores can build up and become toxic. While this will only happen at very high intakes (chronic intake of well over 10,000 IU per day), it is worth keeping in mind, and highlights how a "more of a good thing is better" type attitude can be harmful in the nutrition game.

Commonly used supplements that are, most likely, a waste of your money

BCAAS

BCAAs stands for branch chain amino acids, which, as covered earlier, are a group of 3 amino acids that have particularly anabolic effects (leucine, isoleucine, and valine are the BCAAs). While this may seem like a perfectly sound rationale for using them as a supplement, remember that amino acids are the links that make up protein chains, and provided you get sufficient protein in your diet, you're highly unlikely to benefit from taking BCAAs. Plus, in most instances where you might consider taking BCAAs (e.g. pre- or post-workout), it's far cheaper and beneficial to eat/drink a source of quality protein, like a whey shake, yogurt, or chicken breast.

INDIVIDUAL AMINO ACIDS (LIKE GLUTAMINE)

For the same reason as above, buying individual amino acids, as a means to get hench or shredded, is pretty pointless if you're getting in enough protein. So, save yourself some moolah and go eat a steak.

FAT BURNERS

Most fat burners on the market claim to boost your metabolism, and/or increase the use of body fat for fuel. Thing is, a supplement you'd buy from a high-street store or on a supplement site won't be able to do this to a degree that would have a meaningful effect on your ab pop-ability. Besides, the main active ingredient in most fat burners is caffeine, which is far cheaper and enjoyable as a cup of coffee.

DIET PROTEIN SHAKES

I've never understood diet protein shakes as they typically contain less protein but more carbs and/or fat per 100g than bog standard whey protein powder. Considering protein is the most satiating macronutrient, this just seems backwards to me. So, with that in mind, and given that the supposed fat burning ingredients added to diet shakes have a drop-in-the-ocean-type effect on your fat loss at the very best, you shouldn't waste your money on them.

Key Points

- In the context of a nutritious diet containing a variety of wholefoods, few supplements will impact your results.

- Supplements most likely to be of any benefit include: creatine monohydrate, caffeine, beta alanine, citrulline malate, protein powder, multivitamin/mineral, essential fatty acids/fish oil, vitamin D.

PART 4

MASTERING YOUR NUTRITION STRATEGY AND THE SMART SHRED DIET SYSTEM

Up to this point we've covered the Nutrition Tower, and all the blocks that directly impact its stability, and therefore your results. This next section covers the strategy component of nutrition, and how to put your new-found knowledge into application. So, by the end of Part 4, you'll know exactly how to set up and apply your diet to ensure you don't knock over your Nutrition Tower.

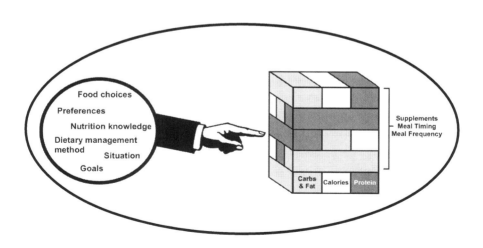

CHAPTER 9

How To Get Abs Without Eating Chicken, Broccoli, And Rice All Day

Talk to most nutrition gurus, and they'll have you believe that if you want a rock-hard set of abs, you've got to say goodbye to all your creamy Ben & Jerry's, gooey doughnuts, and crumbling cookies. On the flipside, you'll be advised to stock your fridge full of Tupperware filled with the likes of chicken, rice, and broccoli; you know, "clean" food.

While there is nothing inherently wrong about this "clean eating" formula, which certainly has worked for lots of guys and girls who have got in to cover model shape, there are some potential diet derailing problems with this sort of approach to dieting, and more often than not, they end up jeopardising your Nutrition Tower somewhere down the line.

In a second, I'll explain exactly why this is the case. However, before I do, I want to make the point that, in the context of this book, I am using the term "clean eating" as a catch-all label for rigid diets that strive for perfection by promoting the consumption of "good" or "clean" foods ONLY, while excluding ALL "bad" or "dirty" foods.

There is nothing wrong with eating foods that are typically classed as "clean"; you know, foods that once walked, swam, grew, or flew. In fact, most of your diet should be made up of this stuff. The issue lies with the rigidity of diets that set certain foods or food groups completely off limits because they're supposedly bad, and that view foods in isolation to the diet as a whole.

And with that said, we can move on to:

THE DIRTY REALITY OF CLEAN EATING: 7 REASONS WHY IT SUCKS

1. Clean Eating Is A Meaningless Term

A vegan's definition of clean eating will be different to that of someone following a paleo diet, which will be different to a ketogenic enthusiast's, and so on. This subjectivity makes "clean eating" very confusing, and blurs the lines of what foods should, and shouldn't, be eaten when trying to strip off fat.

Should you only eat whole grain bread? Should you even be eating bread at all? What about fruit? It's got sugar in it, so does that strike it from the menu? These types of questions are the ones that commonly crop up in the heads of clean eaters. It shouldn't, and needn't be this confusing though.

2. Clean Eating Demonises "Dirty" Foods

Regardless of what is seen as clean or not, the whole demonisation of particular foods and food groups is nonsense; nutrition ain't some sort of religion, and eating strawberry cheesecake vs a bowl of salad isn't a moral decision.

Besides, it misses the bigger picture, and the reality is that the impact of a food on your health and waistline is dependent on how it fits into your diet as a whole. E.g. a snickers bar won't make you sick and fat if the rest of your diet is made up of green stuff, lean meats, and you're not over consuming Calories.

3. Clean Eating Will Most Likely Make You Crave "Dirty" Food Even More

Tell me I can't have something and you bet I'm gonna wanna have it. This is often the case with rigid clean eating, and once you ban certain foods, there's a good chance they'll plague your mind, particularly if they're some of your favourites.

4. Clean Eating Can Make You Feel Guilty As Hell, Increase Your Risk Of Binging, And Make You More Susceptible To Psychological Food Issues

Back in my "clean eating" days, I would refrain from "dirty" food throughout the week, only to flip the switch on the weekend, and enter a no-brownies-spared-pig-out-mode by going ham on all the cookies, pizza, and ice cream I could get my hands on. This pig out only made me feel guiltier than Labrador with the remnants of your roast dinner at its feet, and made me compensate by restricting what I ate extra hard in the days that followed. Let me tell you that this SUCKEDBALLS.com (I urge you to not follow that link …).

It's not just my former self that experienced this though, and the binge-pig out pattern is very common among clean eaters who strive for perfection. It is not healthy from a physiological, and equally as importantly, a psychological standpoint though.

In fact, clean eating is associated with a greater risk of full-blown eating disorders, like anorexia, and has actually been described by nutrition scientists as a new form of eating disorder itself.

105

5. Clean Eating May Increase Your Risk Of Nutrient Deficiencies

This only applies to clean eaters who completely cut out whole food groups like dairy or grains. Without appropriate substitutions, completely eliminating such food groups can create a diet lacking in certain nutrients, and ultimately end up screwing your health.

6. Clean Eating Sucks The Enjoyment Out Of Social Occasions

Often, social occasions with friends, family, and loved ones involve food, which can be a ball-ache if you're following a rigid clean diet. This generally leads to one of two choices being made:

[1] saying screw it to the diet and switching on pig-out-mode

or

[2] missing out on the fun by not getting fully involved in the occasion, or simply not going all together, for fears that it will screw up your diet and make you feel that Labrador-like guilt.

7. Clean Eating May Lead To Suck-ier Results

If the psychological roller-coaster clean eating is often accompanied by isn't enough to convince you of its downfalls, studies have also found that it tends to lead to poorer weight loss results compared to more inclusive and flexible approaches to dieting. This is likely because clean eating is damn hard to stick to, so dieters end up calling it quits early doors, or they simply don't stick to their plan as well.

106

By no means are those points an exhaustive list, and sure, they don't all apply to everyone who ever followed a clean eating type approach to dieting, as for some, eating solely "clean" foods suits them very well. They do highlight some of the major pitfalls of rigid diets though, and for the vast majority of people, I advise a more flexible and inclusive approach to stripping off body fat; it's far more sustainable, and will reduce the chances of your Nutrition Tower toppling over.

Besides, eating nothing but foods that once walked, swam, grew, or flew is completely unnecessary on your quest for abs, and you can get just as good, if not better, results by including the odd bit of "junk" in your diet.

Ben & Jerry's anyone?

ENTER FLEXIBLE DIETING: A LESS RESTRICTIVE WAY TO DIET

Chances are you've come across the term "flexible dieting" before, and may have your own thoughts of what it involves (if not, don't worry; I'm about to give you the low down).

While I don't like to assign names to diets, as it often leads to cult-like followings, the overarching dietary approach I recommend is best described as flexible dieting. My interpretation of what the term means is different to most people's though; so here is my definition that we will be working with in this book:

*Flexible dieting is an overarching mind-set to dieting whereby flexible dieters use their **nutrition knowledge** to make appropriate dietary decisions (i.e. their **food choices**, and the **dietary management method** they use) based on their **goals**, **preferences**, and the **situation** they're in.*

107

Note that this definition refers to flexible dieting as a mind-set, as opposed to a specific diet, which is a very important distinction. Over the next chunk of this section, I'll be dissecting this definition so you fully understand what I, and many of the top nutritionists, fat loss experts, and bodybuilding coaches in the world, consider the best approach to getting a rippling six pack. I'll also go over some of the biggest misconceptions about flexible dieting, which often give it a bad rep.

As highlighted above, flexible dieting incorporates all the components of your Nutrition Strategy mentioned previously. Below is a visual representation of how flexible dieting links them all together.

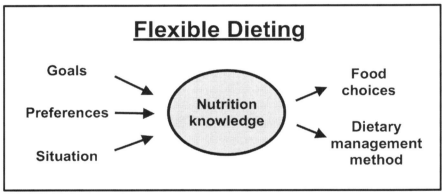

Figure 25.

To explain flexible dieting further, the rest of Part 4 will focus on your **food choices** and **dietary management method**, with reference to how they're affected by your **goals**, **preferences**, and **situation**.

FOOD CHOICES FOR FAT LOSS

As I alluded to above, you don't have to eat a cardboard-like diet to drop the pounds, and doing so may actually screw up your progress in the long run. In fact, a lot of research suggests that chowing down on some custard creams with your cuppa, or Ben & Jerry's post dinner, will improve the results you see in the mirror. This is for a few reasons:

- It helps silence any cravings you have.

- It stops "junk" foods plaguing your mind all day.

- It makes your diet more enjoyable.

- It makes eating out and when on the go easier.

Ultimately, the above means your diet is more likely to fit your lifestyle rather than dictate it, and it will mean you're more likely to stick to it, long term. Given that consistent dietary adherence is key to your progress, choosing to include some "junk" in your diet will, therefore, help you strip the belly fat.

Eat Like A Damn Grownup

So, you can eat all the pancakes, chocolate, and pizza you like then, provided you nail Calories/macros, right?

Well no; not exactly.

I mean, yeah, you could technically get a six pack whilst eating nothing but junk provided you're on point with your Calorie intake, but doing so would make you a dumbass, as you'll just end up sacrificing your health, feeling rubbish, and being hungrier than you would do on a more nutritious diet. So, for those reasons (and because nobody likes a dumbass), eat like a grownup by prioritising the nutritious stuff; you know, lean meats, nuts, seeds, fruit, and veg.

You see, any diet that's followed to improve health, and the body you see in the mirror, should be built on a solid foundation

109

of colourful nutritious foods like fruit and veg. In other words, those "clean" foods I mentioned earlier. Yeah, I know; your Nan could have told you that.

Shopping List Of Nutritious Foods				
Protein Dense Foods	Carb Dense Foods	Fat Dense Foods	Fruit	Veg
Chicken Breast	Brown Rice	Almonds	Apple	Asparagus
Salmon	White Potato	Flax Seed	Nectarine	Celery
Prawns	White Rice	Avocado	Banana	Peas
Sardines	Seeded Bread	Seed Oils	Orange	Carrots
Cottage Cheese	Oats	Butter	Blueberries	Cucumber
Turkey	Wholegrains	Olive Oil	Peach	Pepper
Lean steak	Quinoa	Coconut Oil	Grapes	Broccoli
Mackerel	Beans	Nut Butters	Pear	Green Beans
Egg	Sweet Potato	Dark Chocolate	Kiwi	Courgette
Minced Beef	Lentils	Pecans	Pineapple	Sprouts
Tilapia	Fruits	Walnuts	Berries	Kale
Whey Protein	Parsnips	Oily Fish	Tomato	Spinach
Tuna Steak	Squash	Cashews	Strawberries	Cauliflower
Egg Whites	Milk	Full Fat Dairy	Melon	Onion

Table 5.

These foods provide the nutrients required to maximise your health and energy levels, while minimising your hunger, thus helping you keep your Nutrition Tower standing strong. Again, your Nan could have told you that.

What your Nan probably couldn't tell you is how to hit your flexible dieting sweet spot.

Finding Your Flexible Dieting Sweet Spot

Too much junk, and you'll end up feeling like arse, whereas cutting it out altogether may make your diet fail for the reasons mentioned above (although, if you've no particular desire to eat any cookies or whatever, then obviously, you don't need to; just realise that by the same token, you don't HAVE to completely exclude it).

So, you want to hit the sweet spot, which is dictated by 3 components of your Nutrition Strategy I refer to as The Big 3.

THE BIG 3

HOW YOUR GOALS, PREFERENCES, AND SITUATION DETERMINE YOUR FOOD CHOICES

1. Your goals

If you simply want to cut some fat for a beach break, then you've got a little more wiggle room, and can be more flexible with the foods you choose compared to if you're already pretty lean and looking to shred up even more.

For example, if you're in the depths of contest prep for a bodybuilding show when you're already damn ripped and your Calorie intake is relatively low, you want to be maximising the anti-hunger effects of every bite, which will mean eating proportionally more whole foods and less junk.

2. Your preferences

This is pretty self-explanatory as obviously, your likes and dislikes have a big bearing on the food choices you make and whether you choose to be more or less flexible with your diet by eating more or less "junk".

3. The situation you're in

There are two levels to this:

[1] Think of the first as your *long-term situation*, as it considers where you're currently at on your nutrition journey. For example, if you're trying to dial things in and eat super healthy for one reason or another, you may choose to be less flexible, whereas if you're on autopilot mode or you're super busy with lots going on in your work life, you may be more flexible as realistically you have to include more convenience foods in your diet.

[2] The second level is the *acute situation* you're in. For example, you might be out for the day or at dinner with your friends or family, so choose to be more flexible by eating a little more "junk" than you usually would. On the flipside, midweek when you're following your regular schedule, you can stick to your regular diet of primarily whole foods, so are therefore, less flexible.

Now, while I can't tell you where your flexible dieting sweet spot is because, well, I'm not you, I advise you to:

Limit your intake of highly processed "junk" to a max of 20% of your total Calorie intake.

Obviously there will be the odd day when you pass this threshold, however, you should aim to be consistent with this 20% limit the vast majority of the time, as it will ensure you get in plenty of the nutritious stuff required to feel and perform at your best, and to stave off hunger. So, use this 20% limit as a general rule to stick to whether you're dieting or not.

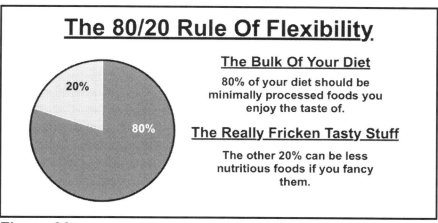

Figure 26.

So, tracking back to Chapter 6 to use Ricky P's Calorie target of 2000 as an example, he would eat up to a max of 400 Calories of whatever he wants.

- That might mean he includes a serving of Honey Nut Cheerios with milk for breakfast (200 Calories), and a Crunchie chocolate bar with his afternoon cuppa (200 Calories).

- Or, it could be that he enjoys a big arse 80g bag of

popcorn (400 Calories), whilst cracking on with an episode of ~~Hannah Montana~~ Game of Thrones.

Either way, so long as his diet is otherwise nutritious, and he doesn't screw up on the Calorie and protein front, 10–20% of "junk" won't kill him or set him back on his road to abs.

However, there is one big Belgian Blue sized caveat here that, if you're not careful, could bulldoze its way through your Nutrition Tower:

Trigger Foods

While this flexible approach means no foods are off limits provided they fit within the guidelines I've given, if you have any trigger foods, you need to cut them out, or manage them appropriately.

What I mean by a trigger food is any food that you're unable to eat in moderation, and one that might trigger one of those pig-out modes I mentioned about earlier. I mean, yeah, eating ice cream and cookies in moderation is great, but sometimes, moderation just isn't possible because some foods are too damn tasty.

So, if there's a food that triggers you to over consume, either:

1. ***Cut it out:*** Exclude it from your diet completely, except for special occasions like birthdays.

Or

2. ***Manage it:*** Find a way to manage your intake of it. For example, I only buy low Calorie tubs of ice cream as, if I start a larger tub, I invariably have to finish it. Because I'm a ~~weirdo~~ legend, I also have the same issue with apples and consequently, I only buy them individually, otherwise, I might devour a whole pack. Dividing foods into sensible portion sizes can also work well.

While we're on the point of exceptions to the rule, if you can't eat certain foods because you're intolerant to them or whatever, then obviously don't. Yeah, that's a really obvious point, but I don't want you getting all sick and that because I failed to mention it in this book.

What If You Do Fall Off The Wagon Though?

Although being flexible with your diet will help manage cravings, and reduce the chances of you having pig out like binges, it would be negligent not to cover how to go about things if you do end up falling off the wagon; we're all human.

Falling off the wagon and over consuming Calories is synonymous to knocking your Nutrition Tower over. Whether it ends up impacting your progress or not comes down to one of two choices you can make if it happens.

Option 1: You don't let a slight overconsumption trigger a pig out.

If you go over your Calorie target slightly because you ate an extra donut, or whatever, but then left it at that, it's no big deal.

This is the ideal "slip up" scenario: you've eaten a little too much, but haven't let it trigger excessive overeating, and have subsequently returned to your regular intake. In other words, you've rebuilt your Nutrition Tower soon after it's fallen. In this instance, you can simply adjust your Calorie intake the next day to account for the slight overconsumption.

For example, if you went 300 Calories over your target one day, you can simply eat 300 Calories less the next day. Limit any adjustment in Calories to 300–400 tops, and refrain from getting into a habit of doing this regularly; it's merely a strategy to use if you slip up slightly on an otherwise consistent diet.

Option 2: You overeat excessively. If you do this, just accept it, and move on.

Going on a food bender because you've veer slightly from your diet is like knocking your Nutrition Tower over and then throwing a hissy fit by chucking the Jenga blocks all over the place. Sure, it might feel good in the moment, but you'll only end up regretting it when time comes to pick up the pieces.

Taking a flexible approach to your diet should go a long way to preventing this form of overeating. However, if you do end up pigging out like this, the best thing to do is just accept it, put it in the past without dwelling on it, and get back to your diet as usual.

I suggest you don't try to compensate in any way for the extra Calories you consumed during your pig out, but just continue your regular diet instead. Yes, it will affect your progress to an extent, but the best thing you can do is just move on and be consistent with your diet again.

DIETARY MANAGEMENT METHODS FOR FAT LOSS

As with the food choices you make, you can also be flexible with the dietary management method you take. By that I mean you don't have to marry yourself to one way of managing your food intake, like tracking your Calories and macronutrients, or using a portion control system.

Which brings me onto one of the biggest flexible dieting misconceptions: it being synonymous with tracking macros and If It Fits Your Macros (IIFYM). It's not, and as I pointed out earlier, flexible dieting is more of a mind-set thing than a set in stone diet. That's not to say that tracking macros isn't a valid management method to dieting, but it's not the only effective one for flexible dieters.

116

In fact, my clients have seen amazing results by using a range of dietary management methods like:

- Macronutrient tracking (i.e. IIFYM)

- Calorie and protein tracking

- Calorie tracking

- Portion control

- Habit based systems (e.g. low carb)

- Ad libitum

Any one of these management methods can work incredibly well for you if it fits "The Big 3": your goals, preferences, and the situation you're in. So, depending on these factors, you can be flexible with the dietary management method you employ.

I want to make these various dietary methods a separate section of this book, so I'm going to explain to you exactly how to choose the right one to maximise your six pack success in Chapter 10.

Key Points

- Striving for perfection by eating solely "clean" foods is a poor way for most people to approach their diet.

- There are no good or bad foods, and what determines the impact of food on your health and waistline is how it fits into your diet as a whole.

- Flexible dieting is about your nutrition/dietary mind-set, and using your nutrition knowledge to make appropriate dietary decisions based on "The Big 3": your goals, preferences, and situation.

- Ensure that at least 80% of your Calories are from nutrient-dense foods the vast majority of the time, leaving up to 20% for a little "junk" if you'd like.

- Manage any trigger foods appropriately. You may need to cut them out of your diet.

- If you fall off the wagon by overeating a little (by 300–400 Calories or so), compensate by eating fewer the next day. If you overeat by a lot, don't try to compensate for it the next day; just accept it, move on, and get back to your dieting plan of action.

- There is no single approach to dieting that works for everyone; it's about finding the one that suits you personally.

CHAPTER 10

How To Choose The Right Dietary Management Method: The 6 Step Smart Shred Diet System

In a minute I'll go over the Smart Shred Diet System; a tried and tested science-based fat loss system that my clients have used to get into incredible shape. This system will tell you exactly what to do to ensure you start shredding fat from the off, and will take you through a structured process towards optimising your diet and Nutrition Strategy.

Figure 27 shows a brief overview to give context to the first part of this chapter.

Don't worry about its ins and outs just yet; I'll explain it in more detail in a minute. However, before I do, we're going to go through the 5 main management methods I recommend when dieting (well, 5½), as it provides the background required to fully appreciate the system.

Although it's quite self-explanatory, what I mean by "dietary management method" is a method that's used to control different variables – or Jenga blocks – of your diet, like your Calories, protein, and carbs/fat. There are a bazillion of these methods out there in the dieting world, however, regardless of the specific one used, they all control Calories in one way or another, whether it's through a pseudo system, like tracking syns, or by counting them directly.

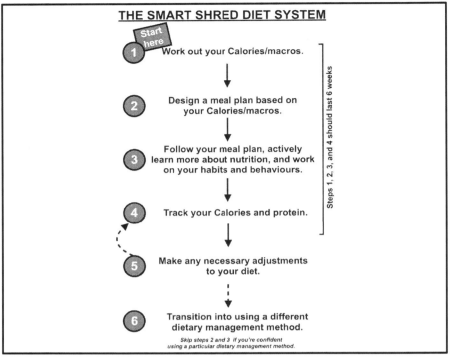

Figure 27.

The dietary management methods recommended here are the ones that I have found to be most effective for attaining a chiselled body with ripped abs. For each method, I'll explain what it is and how to implement it, before going into the pros and cons of each, and what contexts they're best suited to. So, without further ado, let's crack on.

1. MACRO TRACKING

This is the classic IIFYM type method, whereby you track your Calorie and macronutrient (protein, carbs, fat) intake using an app like MyFitnessPal.* It's very simple, in that all you have to

---

Visit www.tommycole.co.uk/bookbonuscontent for a MyFitnessPal tutorial.

do is download the app and then plug in every Calorie containing food/drink you consume. Remember that macros are what provide you with Calories, so if you hit your macros as closely as possible, you'll nail your Calorie target by default.

I say hit your macros as closely as possible, but there's no need to get all neurotic about it because the reality is that the nutritional content shown on food labels/databases won't be 100% accurate for the specific food you're eating. For example, two sirloin steaks weighing in at 200g will inevitably vary slightly in the amount of fat and other nutrients they contain. Besides, digestion isn't a perfect process, so the amount of energy or a given macro your body actually absorbs from the food you eat, can vary. For these reasons – and for the sake of your sanity – I advise that you aim to be within[*]:

- **20g of your protein and carb targets;**

- **10g of your fat target;**

- **and 100 Calories of your Calorie target.**

Here's an example of how to set this up:

Calories/Macros	Calculated Target	Range To Be Within
Calories	2000	1900–2100
Protein	160g	140–180g
Fat	80g	70–90g
Carbs	160g	140–180g

Table 6.

---

[*]*If you're looking to compete in bodybuilding or a physique competition, then you might want to make the ranges tighter. So +/- 10g for protein and carbs, 5g for fat, and the same +/- 100 for Calories.*

2. CALORIE AND PROTEIN TRACKING

You know I said that Calories and protein are the two nutrition variables that will have the greatest impact on your fat loss?

Well, this means that if you can't be arsed to be bang on with all your macros, you can just prioritise the more important factors, and still see incredible progress.

You implement this method in the same way as full-blown Calorie and macro tracking, but instead of trying to hit your fat and carb targets within those +/- 10–20g ranges mentioned above, you just let carbs and fat fill in the remaining Calories after hitting protein, without fussing over specific amounts of either.

So you consistently hit your Calorie and protein targets, but one day, you might have a higher carb to fat ratio, and the next might be the opposite and higher in fat than carbs.

This is the method I advise the majority of committed dieters to follow for sculpting a ripped body.

3. CALORIE TRACKING

Yup, you guessed it; this is like the above, but you just hit your Calorie target without paying much attention to your macros, as your Calorie intake is the big dog of fat loss nutrition.

Again, I advise you use the +/- 100 Calorie range to see the best results.

3 ½. MEAL PLANS: A TOOL TO HIT YOUR CALORIE AND/OR MACRO TARGETS

While rigid meal plans do work great for some people, I don't tend to advise the exclusive use of them, particularly if it's without a background understanding of Calories, macronutrients, and nutrition in general. This is because rigid plans can leave dieters without knowing how to approach their nutrition once they've finished their fat loss diet; kind of like how you can blindly follow a satnav and consequently have no idea where to go if its battery dies.

Personally, I prefer to use meal plans as a guidance tool (as opposed to a rigid plan) and something to build upon. For example, I often provide clients with sample meal plans to show what certain Calorie/macro targets might look like from a food perspective. In fact, I advise you to plan out at least some of your meals, particularly if all this talk of Calorie and macro tracking is new to you (more on exactly how I suggest you do this in a minute). Just make sure you understand that you don't HAVE to rigidly stick to them, there is no single meal plan that is above and beyond all others, and they're simply a tool you can use to plan out and hit given Calorie/macro targets.

How To Design Your Meal Plan

I've included an example 7-day meal plan at the end of this chapter, which you can also download at www.tommycole.co.uk/bookbonuscontent. It will work well for most guys as a starting point, but needs personalisation.

To plan out meals yourself, simply take the Calorie/macro targets you worked out above, and put together foods and meals that hit them. If you're stuck for ideas, visit www.eatthismuch.com; this site does all the hard work for you by taking your Calorie/macro targets and putting together a free meal plan for you instantly. Alternatively, use Table 5 in Chapter 9 as guidance, and enter meals into MyFitnessPal to tally up the Calories/macros so they hit your targets. This meal planning takes time initially, but it's a valuable process on your nutrition journey.

4. PORTION CONTROL

Here, we're moving away from direct Calorie/macro counting and instead are using our hands as a guide to control portion sizes of the various macronutrients. You see, whilst many foods contain a mix of the different macronutrients, most tend to be higher in one than the other. For example, potatoes are mostly carbs, chicken breast is mostly protein, and avocados are primarily fat; as can be seen in the Venn diagram below.

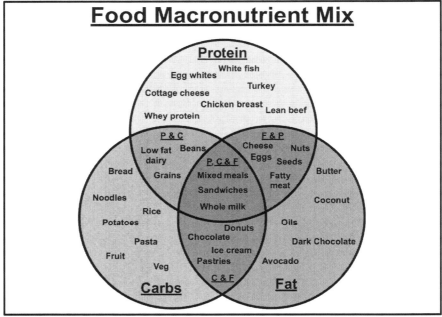

Figure 28.

So, aiming for a certain number of portions of the various macronutrients works as a crude way to track your macros, and therefore, Calories.

As For Portion Control Guidelines, Follow This 3-Step System

Step 1

Use Table 7 as a reference for what an individual portion of protein, fat, and carbohydrate equates to.

Step 2

Take the same macronutrient calculations explained above in "Macro tracking" and convert this into portions by using the info in the table.*

So, if your daily carb target were 200g, that's 5 fist portions, as each fist equates to around 40g of carbs. Expanding on this example with a hypothetical intake of 200g carbs, 150g protein, 60g fat:

$$200g \text{ carbs} = 5 \text{ fist portions } (200 \div 40)$$
$$150g \text{ protein} = 5 \text{ fist portions } (150 \div 30)$$
$$60g \text{ fat} = 4 \text{ thumb portions } (60 \div 15)$$

Step 3

Now, you've got daily portion targets. Either:

[1] divide this up into portions to have per meal.

For portion control, consider non-starchy vegetables – like leafy greens – as separate to your carbohydrate portions, and aim for 1–2 veg portions per meal. Fruit tends to be more carb dense than vegetables, so factor them into your carb portions.

So, using the same example, your meals might look like this:

Breakfast = 1 portion carbs, 1 portion protein, 1 portion fat
Lunch = 2 portion carbs, 2 portion protein, 1 portion fat
Dinner = 2 portion carbs, 2 portion protein, 2 portion fat

Or *[2]* tally up your portions as you go, throughout the day, like this:

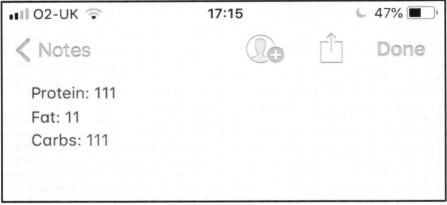

Figure 29.

Ultimately, each of these two methods will end up with you eating the same number of portions over the course of the day; so, whichever you choose just depends on your preference.

As with all other dietary management methods, like macro tracking, the initial calculations and resulting portion targets are just a starting point, and it's up to you to adjust them after a couple of weeks if necessary. So, if you're not losing weight, you could take away a portion or two of carbs or fat, for example.

Macronutrient	What Equates To 1 Portion	What This Looks Like
Carbohydrate Dense Food	1 closed fist Equal to around 40g of carbs	
Protein Dense Food	1 closed fist Equal to around 30g of protein	
Fat Dense Food	1 thumb Equal to around 15g of fat (or 1 tbsp oil)	

Table 7.

5. HABIT BASED

As the term suggests, habit based dieting involves focusing on consistent eating patterns and nailing certain dietary behaviours that are conducive towards achieving your goals. The particular habits you focus on will be quite individualised, but for this fat loss system, the habits to implement are as follows.

Fat Loss Habits

- Read food labels to estimate your Calorie intake and to roughly hit your Calorie needs.

- Eat 3 meals per day and 1 protein based snack. So breakfast, lunch, dinner, and a floating snack to go in whenever you'd like.

- Make sure each meal contains a portion of protein, and two portions of veg.

- Eat at the same time of the day, every day.

- The two meals around your training should contain 1–2 portions of starchy carbs. So if you train in the afternoon, these meals would be lunch and dinner.

- Drink 2–3l of fluid.

- Sit down at a table when eating, without any distractions like the TV.

- Eat slowly, chew each mouthful 10–20 times, and savour the taste of your food.

- Remove Calorie dense foods from your living environment. Obviously this isn't always possible if they don't belong to you, but even putting junk foods away in a cupboard can help; out of sight, out of mind and all.

Regardless of whether you're tracking macros, Calories, or whatever else, I recommend the above habits, particularly if you don't have a great deal of structure to your current, pre shred diet. In the Smart Shred Diet System, there's a period of time to work on introducing habits, of which these are great ones to go with.

Track Calories/Macros Initially To Tune Your Habits

This habit based method is most effective for people who already have a solid grasp on nutrition and portion sizing. In fact, I find that a period of macro or Calorie tracking prior to starting a habit based method works well, as it helps tune your habitual eating patterns and portions so that they're in line with your goals.

For the same reasons, it's also a good idea to track Calories or macros periodically throughout your diet for a few days or a week at a time, even if you are primarily using a different dietary management method, like habit based dieting; it works as a means to tune your diet and stay on track.

Combine Habits With Dietary Rules

Also, while these habits will help drive fat loss, I suggest that they're used in combo with dietary rules, as such rules allow for greater control, tend to make you eat less, and ultimately help ensure you drop into a Calorie deficit by default.

Commonly implemented rules that help drive fat loss when using a habit based method include:

- Intermittent fasting

- Low carb dieting

- Low fat dieting

- "Clean eating"

Yeah, yeah; I know that might seem pretty contradictory to what I said earlier in that you needn't be overly rigid with your diet, and don't have to eat clean, cut out carbs, fat, or whatever else, to see results. But there is a trade-off you must consider when using less precise methods, like habit based dieting, and ultimately, you'll probably have to be more rigid with your diet to optimise your progress using this method; it will help you maintain sufficient control of your diet and ultimately, your total Calorie intake.

And this gives a good Segway to start discussing the pros/cons of each method, and how to choose the right one for you.

DIETARY PRECISION AND FLEXIBILITY

With all the dietary management methods above, there are pros and cons; full blown macro tracking gives you the tightest control over your diet, but some find logging their food in an app a pain in the arse (this pain in the arse-ness of tracking tends to disappear after a week or so of getting used to it though). On the flipside, portion control doesn't require you to track using an app, however, you can't be as precise, which might impact progress and means you have to be a little stricter with the foods you consume.

So, the different dietary management methods fall onto a precision continuum, with Calorie and macro counting at the more precise end, and habit based dieting being less precise. Because of this, the degree of flexibility you can get away with varies from one method to another.

For example, because you're closely tracking what goes in your gob when counting Calories and/or macros, you can afford to be a little more flexible, both with your eating patterns and the foods you consume (obviously while sticking to the "Eat Like A Damn Grownup" guidelines that is).

With the less precise methods, you're relying more on hunger levels to control your food intake, and you're also not as aware of the Calories you're consuming. This means you'll need to stick to a more consistent dietary structure, and be more mindful of what you consume. So, with all that in mind, we're going to come back to The Big 3, and how they determine the right method for you.

THE BIG 3

HOW YOUR GOALS, PREFERENCES, AND SITUATION DETERMINE YOUR DIETARY MANAGEMENT METHOD

1. Goals

If you're looking to get really shredded, then you're best off sticking to the more precise methods of tracking. The same can be said if you have a tight and important deadline to get in shape for, like a big photo shoot, and/or if you want to maximise your performance and results.

---

2. Preferences

Self-explanatory, and if you dislike tracking macros or whatever else, you may be more suited to another method.

3. Situation

Again, this can be broken down into your long term and acute situation.

[1] Your *long term situation* accounts for what's going on in your life at the time, like if you've got a family to feed, or whether you've got a hectic work schedule, which may both make Calorie/macro tracking more difficult. Conversely, after a holiday, where you've taken an ad libitum or habit based method, you may transition back into a more precise tracking method, like Calorie counting. Your long term situation also accounts for where you are on your nutrition journey: do you have prior macro tracking experience? What's your level of nutrition knowledge? Do you have a structure to your diet and meals already? Or, are you starting from scratch, with no previous structure and a diet of pizza, chips, and bagels? These are all factors to consider, and if you feel you have little dieting experience and/or knowledge, then jumping in at the deep end, with full blown macro tracking, might be a bit much. On the flipside, you may find the precision of macro tracking helps kick you off, and keeps you accountable; it really depends on you as an individual, and you need to consider these Big 3 factors together, before making a decision.

[2] The *acute situation* you're in may change the method you choose to use for a number of reasons too. For example, if you're out for a meal with your partner, you may switch from tracking macros to just Calories, or you may choose to estimate portion sizes instead. You might also simply want a day off from tracking macros and/or Calories; so use a less precise method for a day or so.

This is where having a flexible approach to dieting comes into its own because you're able to make your diet fit your lifestyle, rather than it being the other way around. It also means you're able to maintain some level of control over your diet, regardless of the situation.

So, there is no right or wrong dietary management method to use. Rather, there are various methods that sit on a precision spectrum, and it's up to you to choose which is right for you, depending on The Big 3 factors.

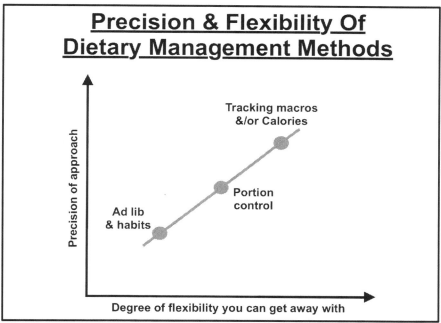

Figure 30.

With all that said, I do recommend a period of Calorie and/or macro tracking initially, which is for a number of reasons:

- It teaches you so much about what is in the food you consume.

135

- It will boost your awareness of how much you actually eat (this is a big one as most people suck at estimating how many Calories they eat).

- Using a food diary app helps keep you accountable.

- It is a precise method of dieting and consequently, will help maximise your progress early doors, which will help keep you motivated to play out the rest of your diet.

- It helps ingrain dietary habits.

- It sets you up for transitioning into less precise methods, like portion control, as you'll know how much of what to eat to see progress.

- It will make you better at "eyeballing" portion sizes.

In fact, while it's important to consider all of the above and select the right dietary management method for you, I recommend you follow the 6 Step Smart Shred Diet System I outline on the next page, starting at step 1 and then moving on to 2 or 4, depending on your nutrition knowledge and experience.

When to move from step 1 to step 2

If you're sat there at all unsure about what level your nutrition knowledge and experience is at, then it's best to consider yourself a beginner and follow the system in its entirety by going from step 1 to 2.

When to move from step 1 to step 4

If you're experienced with using a particular method, you can skip steps 2 and 3, going straight to step 4, where you focus on tracking Calories and protein. Also, if you're confident to go without using a meal plan, you don't necessarily need one as guidance. I advise you to plan at least some meals out though.

THE 6 STEP SMART SHRED DIET SYSTEM

1. *Set Your Nutrition Targets:* Work out your Calorie and macronutrient targets.

2. *Design Your Meal Plan:* Design a meal plan based on these targets. Take into account your personal preferences, and habitual eating patterns, and make sure your plan spans at least, 3–4 days, so you have plenty of options to select from (use www.eatthismuch.com to plan it out, and see the example below, which you can download at www.tommycole.co.uk/bookbonuscontent).

3. *Follow Your Meal Plan:* Follow your meal plan, while actively learning more about nutrition, your diet, and the foods you eat. This is the time to start reading food labels, noting how certain foods contribute to your fullness, and modifying your dietary and lifestyle habits so they're conducive to your goals (e.g. cooking more often, prepping meals, eating at the dinner table as opposed to in front of the TV etc). You can track with MyFitnessPal a little during this stage, but it's not a necessary part of the system until step 4. Dedicate a minimum of <u>2 weeks</u> to step 3.

4. *Track Whilst Using Your Meal Plan:* Start tracking your Calorie and protein intake while continuing to use your meal plan as guidance. Don't worry about trying to hit specific targets for carbs and fat; just let them fall into place as you focus on Calories and protein. You may need to stick fairly tightly to your meal plan at the beginning, but the goal is to become more flexible by incorporating more meals outside of your plan, as you gain experience tracking.

5. ***Adjust Your Nutrition Targets If Needed:*** Once you've followed this process for a few weeks (I suggest <u>4 weeks at step 4 minimum</u>), you will have gained a much greater understanding of nutrition, and how your body responds to your diet and various aspects of nutrition. You will also have plenty of data (weight recordings, Calorie intake etc) that you can use to adjust things if needs be. If you do adjust anything (e.g. you lower Calorie intake), give any changes 2 more weeks of tracking before reassessing and moving on to step 6.

6. ***Transition If You're Confident:*** Move away from the strict use of your meal plan. This is the point where you decide whether to continue to track your Calorie and protein intake, or transition into a different dietary management method if you're confident (denoted by the dashed arrows in Figure 27). This is the stage where you consider all the possible options and which one will suit you best, based on The Big 3.

If you're experienced with one method and are confident about using it, skip steps 2, and 3, and move straight to 4 where you track Calories and protein initially for the reasons I highlighted earlier.

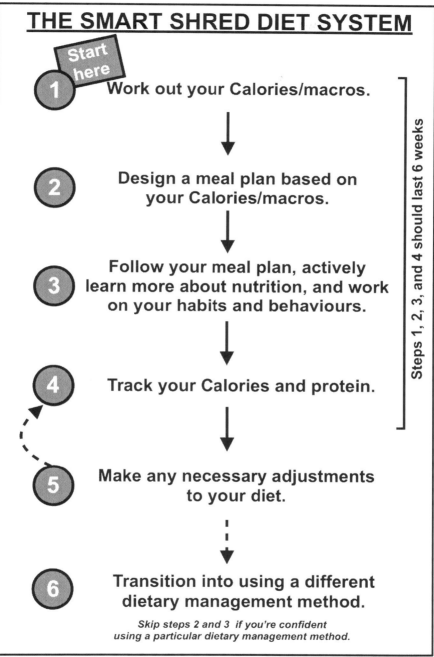

Figure 27.

Key Points

- There are many effective management methods to dieting.

- The most effective include tracking macronutrients, tracking Calories, portion control, and habit based methods.

- Meal plans are a great tool to help you hit your nutrition targets, but are best used alongside other methods to prevent over reliance on them.

- Your goals, preferences, and situation determine the best dietary management method for you.

- An initial phase of tracking Calories and/or macronutrients will help set you up for success, even if you don't use tracking as your main method to dieting.

- The Smart Shred Diet System is a tried and tested scientific approach to dieting that will help maximise fat loss and your transformation progress.

Meal Plan Example

	Breakfast	Lunch	Dinner	Snack
Day 1	Eggs on toast: 3 eggs, 2 slices of toast, 1 tsp olive oil, 1 tbsp ketchup	Chicken wrap: 200g grilled chicken breast, half avocado, handful lettuce, 100g salsa, 1 wrap	Cottage pie: 200g potato, 200g 5% minced beef, 200g chopped tomatoes, 1 carrot, 1 onion, handful mushrooms, half tsp marmite, salt/pepper, half teaspoon each of cumin, paprika, chilli powder, 1 tsp butter to cook	Apple, protein shake (30g powder with water)
Day 2	Proats: 60g oats cooked with water, 30g whey protein, banana	Jacket potato: medium potato with leftover cottage pie filling, served with mixed salad, cucumber and cherry tomatoes	Ham, egg and chips: 150g ham, 2 eggs, 200g potato chopped into chips and baked in 1 tsp olive oil, 1 tbsp ketchup	250g high protein yogurt (e.g. Fage, Skyre) with handful of berries
Day 3	Omelette: 3 eggs, 20g light cheddar cheese, handful mushrooms, 1 tbsp ketchup	Tuna bun: 1 tin tuna, 1 tbsp BBQ sauce, burger bun, side salad of tomatoes and mixed leaves	Beef burrito: 200g 5% minced beef, 1 red pepper, 1 onion, lettuce, 2 wraps, 200g salsa, half avocado	2 rice cakes topped with 50g cottage cheese and 50g ham
Day 4	Protein pancake: 1 egg, 30g protein powder, 1 banana, 15g oats, 1 tsp olive oil to cook, handful berries, 1 tbsp reduced sugar jam	Turkey sandwich: 150g turkey breast, 1 tbsp cranberry sauce, 1 tbsp light cream cheese, lettuce, 2 slices wholemeal bread	Chicken stir fry: 200g chicken breast, 1 onion, handful mushrooms, handful mangetout, handful green beans, 1 chopped garlic clove, half teaspoon chopped ginger, 1 tbsp soy sauce, 1 tsp rice wine vinegar, 150g pre-cooked noodles	25g nuts (e.g. cashews, almonds, walnuts)

142

Day 5	Yogurt: 250g high protein yogurt, apple, sweetener, cinnamon	Salad: 120g diced chicken, cherry tomatoes, shredded carrot, half avocado, couple handfuls of mixed salad, dress with 1 tsp olive oil and balsamic	Steak: 200g lean steak, 1 tsp butter to cook, 200g baked sweet potato, 1 shredded carrot and 1 shredded courgette dressed in juice of 1 lime, 1 tbsp soy sauce and sprinkle of chopped fresh coriander	Protein bar
Day 6	Scrambled egg: 3 eggs, 1 tsp butter to cook, 2 slices of toast, handful spinach, handful cherry tomatoes, 1 tbsp ketchup or bbq sauce	Honey mustard salad: 1 baked cod fillet, 2 handfuls mixed salad, half red onion, handful cherry tomatoes, handful chopped cucumber, half red pepper, dressing (1 tsp runny honey, 1 tsp french mustard, 1 tsp balsamic vinegar, 1 tsp olive oil)	Baked salmon fillet cooked with lemon juice and garlic, jacket potato and a couple of handfuls of mixed salad and steamed beetroot, dressed with balsamic vinegar and 1 tsp olive oil	Protein shake (30g powder), orange
Day 7	Cereal and shake: 50g of coco pops, 200ml semi skimmed milk, protein shake (30g powder)	Tuna sandwich: 1 tin tuna, 1 tbsp light mayo, handful sweetcorn, 2 slices of wholemeal bread, cucumber sticks	Vegetarian coconut curry: 200g butternut squash, half onion, 1 garlic clove, 1 tsp coconut oil to cook, half can low fat coconut milk, half can lentils, half tsp turmeric, half tsp cumin, sprinkle of chopped fresh coriander, salt/pepper, cauliflower rice	250g high protein yogurt (eg: fage, skyre) with pear

Table 8.

PART 5

THE LOOSE ENDS

Throughout this book, I've hinted at a few topics that weren't covered in full at the time because I wanted to cover other things first. So this section ties up some loose ends from prior sections of the book by giving them the detailed breakdown they deserve.

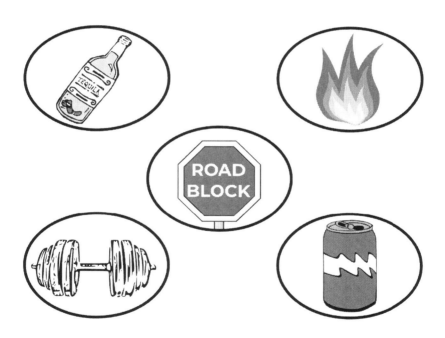

CHAPTER 11

Fluid, The Truth About Sweeteners, And Drinking Alcohol When Dieting

It goes without saying that being hydrated and drinking sufficient fluid is damn important for, well, pretty much everything, and if you don't stay hydrated, then you're doing your body, health, and performance a disservice.

SETTING FLUID TARGETS

A really simple fluid target to aim for is:

1–1.5 ml per Calorie consumed.

I like this method, as it will indirectly scale with your activity level, given that you'll require more Calories the more active you are. Going by this target, most should drink in the region of 2–4l per day. I also suggest you get in roughly a pints worth of water, in the two hours before exercise.

As for what contributes to your hydration level, pretty much anything bar alcohol goes. Yes, that means your teas, coffees, and diet drinks will help hydrate you, which goes against what many believe. With that said, it is advisable to get most of your fluid needs from water, and be wary of overdoing the caffeinated and diet drinks. In other words, be an adult about it; despite diet drinks and teas/coffees being absolutely fine in moderate amounts, clearly drinking nothing but them is a dumbass thing to do from a health perspective.

So, Diet Drinks And Artificial Sweeteners Are Fine Then?

Yes; I know they're often demonised, but this is merely because the science that has linked them to any sort of ill health effect has been blown way out of proportion. Here's a breakdown based on what the body of science currently says:

- There is research that has shown some sweeteners to cause health issues (mostly in rats), such as impacting gut bacteria.

- Said research generally uses very large doses of sweeteners that no normal person would ever come close to consuming, let alone those of us who are conscious about our health.

- The accepted daily intake of aspartame (one of the most common sweeteners used) is equivalent to around 20 cans of diet coke.

- Obviously, you shouldn't drink that much anyway, but like I said, no sensible person would.

- A can or so per day is more than likely to have absolutely no ill health effects, and if it's replacing a sugary drink, it will be a positive change.

- Finally, context is key: do you think the odd diet drink will ruin your health if your diet is full of fruit, veg, and all that good stuff? If you answered yes, then I have failed you as your logic fostering nutritionist; and for that, I sincerely apologise. If you answered no, then go forth and have a Pepsi Max.

148

So, again, it comes down to being an adult about it, and not overdoing the stuff. In reality, having the occasional diet drink is fine, and if it replaces a Calorie containing one, then it's a sensible substitution as drinking your Calories is something I generally advise against, particularly when dieting.

So don't drink your Calories.

This is because drinks don't have the same filling effect as food, so you're much better off eating as many of your Calories as possible.

While, for many, swapping out a regular Coke or Fanta for the diet alternative won't come as a struggle, when it comes to beer, wine, and other alcoholic drinks, scrapping them completely when dieting may not be realistic.

Don't you worry yourself, though, as I'll cover the mistake inducing, fun forging, jolly juice that is alcohol next.

ALCOHOL

I'm not going to pretend that drinking alcohol won't impact your results, particularly if you drink heavily on the weekend or when out with friends, but you certainly can include some alcohol in your diet and still get abs.

Plus, provided you're somewhat strategic with your drinking and don't go washing the booze down with 3 cheeseburgers, French fries, and a 20 pack of nugs in the early hours of the morning (we're all guilty of this at some point), you can get drunk while stripping body fat too.

By no means am I condoning excessive drinking; I'm just being real here, as lots of us enjoy the odd drinking sesh.

So, Here's The Deal With Alcohol

First off, like protein, carbs, and fat, alcohol (ethanol) is a macronutrient. The thing with alcohol is that our body freaks the hell out when we consume it; so it goes straight to the front of the metabolism line. By that, I mean that fat, carb, and protein metabolism (burning) gets put on the back burner, as our body prioritises dealing with alcohol. This is because, unlike fat, carbs, and protein, our bodies can't store alcohol; so if it's not given all the attention, it ends up hanging around for too long and stirs up trouble, as its metabolic by-product (acetate) is toxic. So, our bodies shut down fat burning to deal with the alcohol, meaning your early morning 20 pack of nugs is more likely to be stored as fat when getting drunk.

Given that alcohol is one of the macros, it also provides 7 Calories per gram. So, while no one goes around drinking pure alcohol, 10g of the stuff racks in at 70 Calories. That's roughly the amount of alcohol in a standard shot of spirit, like vodka or tequila, which therefore, add up to around 70–100 Calories each.

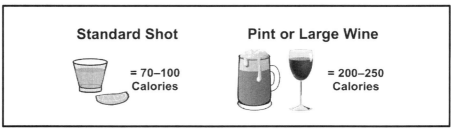

Standard Shot = 70–100 Calories

Pint or Large Wine = 200–250 Calories

Figure 31.

Other alcoholic drinks have lots of other Calorie containing stuff added to them (like sugar), and spirits are usually drunk in combo with Calorie containing mixers, like Coke and tonic. For example, a standard pint of beer racks in at around 220 Calories, an espresso martini contains in the region of 300 Calories, and a single vodka and Coke is 120.

So, as you can see, it's easy to quickly gulp down a high Calorie count from a few drinks or a night out. As I mentioned earlier, that doesn't mean you need to completely forego drinking when you're trying to strip off pounds though.

And with all that in mind, we can get into the practical stuff.

How To Incorporate Alcohol Into Your Diet: 5 Tips

1. Learn to say no

If you've got a goal to lose fat then accept that there will be some degree of sacrifice you have to make. So, ideally minimise the amount of alcohol you drink when dieting, and consider if you genuinely want to drink when in a potential boozing situation, whether it be a casual beer with dinner or night out with friends. In social situations, you might feel pressure to drink, but if you don't actually want a beer, glass of wine, or whatever, just be an adult about it and say no (this also applies when offered stuff like cake; if you genuinely don't want it for one reason or another, just adult-up and say no).

2. Eat fewer Calories in the day

If you do want to drink, then prepare for it earlier on in the day by eating fewer Calories. Do this by consuming less fat (or carbs) as opposed to reducing protein intake. How you go about this is to firstly work out how many Calories are in what you plan to drink. Then take this Calorie target, and divide it by 9 (or 4 for carbs). The result you get is the number of grams you need to take off your fat (or carb) target.

E.g. if you're having a 220 Calorie pint of beer, consume 25g less fat.

It's best to take the Calories away from fat as they're the most likely to be stored as body fat when drinking, but this isn't a huge deal, so if you'd prefer, take it from your carb target, or just focus on your overall Calorie target instead.

3. Eat mostly protein, fruit, and veg in the day

You're best off doing the maths as above and tracking where possible, but if you'd rather not track, then focus primarily on consuming protein dense foods, and low-Calorie stuff like fruit and veg earlier on in the day; this will give you a good Calorie buffer for a few drinks. Also, make sure you stay hydrated throughout the day and night as I will help with fullness and your head the following day.

4. Be smart with your choice of drink

Choose lower Calorie drinks and if having a mixer, make it a diet/zero Calorie one. On a quantity of alcohol per Calorie basis, spirits, with or without a diet mixer, are the best option, whereas beers and cocktails are pretty sucky (you can find a drinks comparison resource in the bonus content).

Personally, if I'm having more than a couple, my go-to drinks are tequila and diet lemonade, or vodka and diet coke. If I'm having a casual beer, then I'd rather sacrifice some Calories, and have a quality Belgian beer.

5. Don't round off your night with a takeaway

When we drink alcohol, our dietary restraint is inhibited, which means we're far more likely to down a family bucket of chicken, and consequently triple our day's Calorie intake. This is where you can do some major damage to your quest for abs, as you can easily counteract a hard week of dieting with an early morning pig out.

I actually suggest you get any tempting foods out of sight and reach if possible. So if you know you'll be out late drinking one night, don't leave a pack of cookies hanging around in the kitchen ready to be engulfed when you arrive back home. This is a good rule to carry over to your lifestyle in general as it will make you less likely to reach for an unnecessary snack.

Key Points

- Aim for 1–1.5ml of fluid per Calorie consumed. For most that's 2–4l per day.

- Minimise any Calorie consumption from drinks.

- Alcohol is a macronutrient and contains 7 Calories per gram.

- Alcoholic drinks contain lots of Calories.

- Drinking alcohol lowers your ability to resist tempting foods.

- Drinking lots of alcohol is clearly unhealthy and will impact your results.

- You can incorporate alcohol into your diet and still lose fat though.

- To do this: choose lower Calorie drinks, avoid the post drinking takeaway, and consume fewer Calories in the day, with most coming from protein and fruit/veg.

CHAPTER 12

Overcoming A Plateau

Now that we've covered the Nutrition Tower in its entirety, and you've got a structured system to strip off fat (i.e. The Smart Shred Diet System), we're going to fast-forward to a few months down the line: you've followed the system, dialed in your diet, started shifting pounds, and you're slowly uncovering more definition, week by week.

After a while, your progress starts to slow a little though, and you end up hitting a roadblock in your diet: the dreaded weight loss plateau.

If you start your diet with a lot of weight to lose, then there's a good chance you'll come to such a plateau point somewhere along your dieting timeline. For many unprepared dieters, this point prompts an outbreak of Google activity, which may result in said dieter considering all manner of approaches to re-ignite fat loss:

- Popping fat burners.

- Gulping down diet teas and drinks.

- Drastically switching up meal frequency.

These are all things past clients of mine had tried prior to working with me.

THEY.DID.NOT.WORK. Which I'd hope comes as no surprise to you.

Fortunately, you won't make these mistakes though, as by now you should have a solid grasp on the fundamentals of fat loss. So, you'll understand that these sorts of approaches are ineffective in and of themselves, and that whatever it is you do, it must ultimately result in you consuming fewer Calories than you expend, over a prolonged period of time.

In this chapter, I'm going to be expanding on this by breaking down the most effective strategies to re-spark fat loss during a plateau. However, before all that, I'll cover why it is they happen.

WHY DOES FAT LOSS SOMETIMES STALL?

Ultimately, our bodies are built to survive, and consequently, they're very adaptable. Due to this adaptability, our bodies fight against our six-pack endeavours to some degree.

You see, when food wasn't as available as it is today, we would go long periods of time on a pretty frugal number of Calories and were, therefore, at real danger of dying from starvation as we got skinnier. As a means to stretch these frugal Calories as far as possible and save us from starvation, our bodies would reduce the amount of Calories we required/burnt.

Fast forward to the modern day, and despite us being at virtually no danger of starvation with today's food availability, our bodies still retain this adaptability.

What sparks this change in energy expenditure is body fat levels. So, when we have a high amount of body fat, this tells us that we've got lots of energy available, so we become less efficient and burn more Calories. On the flip side, when our abs are starting to pop, our low level of body fat signals to our body that stores are low, so we become more efficient at burning Calories.

It's a little like how small cars, like my sub 1 litre Peugeot 107, are typically more efficient at burning fuel than big arse ones, like a Range Rover; the smaller your body fat stores, the more efficient you are at burning the fuel (Calories) you put into your body.

So, over the course of your diet, as you lose fat, you'll gradually start burning fewer Calories.

If you track back to Chapter 4 where I covered the different components of metabolism, you'll remember that we can break it down into 4 categories: basal metabolic rate (BMR), thermic effect of feeding (TEF), exercise activity thermogenesis (EAT), and non-exercise activity thermogenesis (NEAT).

Here Is How They Change As You Lose Weight And Body Fat

- **BMR:** hormonal changes decrease the number of Calories you burn at rest. Plus, it's possible you'll lose some muscle as you diet. Because both muscle and body fat burn Calories, as you lose quantities of these tissues you burn fewer Calories. Together, these changes might account for a drop of up to 15–20%. So, at the upper end, a large person who's lost lots of weight might burn around 300–400 fewer Calories at complete rest.

- **TEF:** As you eat less food, you burn fewer Calories for digestion.

- **EAT:** As your diet goes on, your performance in the gym may drop, and you might feel more lethargic when doing exercise, ultimately leading to fewer Calories being burnt.

- **NEAT:** We subconsciously get lazier as we lose fat, and end up standing, fidgeting, and generally moving less. On the flipside, we start sitting, slouching, and being sloth-like more. The degree to which we morph into a sloth varies greatly between people, so some might have a large drop in Calorie burn due to changes in NEAT, whereas others might have very little. Because we carry less weight around as our diet progresses, we also burn fewer Calories during activity for the simple fact that our muscles don't have to work as hard.

Changes in EAT and NEAT are what tend to account for the greatest drop in energy expenditure over the course of a diet, and while the adaptations to BMR (e.g. hormonal changes) do reduce our Calorie burn, the extent to which they do is often exaggerated greatly, with many Gurus harping on about starvation mode[*] and massive drops in BMR causing plateaus, or even fat gain, whilst eating sub 1000 Calories. Such extreme cases can pretty much always be explained by misreporting of Calorie intake, be it intentional or not.

What all this sciency stuff means is that you gradually burn fewer Calories as you diet, and if your Calorie intake stays the same, eventually your Calorie expenditure will match your intake. As a result, you hit a weight loss plateau, and need to make a change to fire up fat loss once again.

HOW TO RE-IGNITE FAT LOSS

First off, you need to be sure that it's a legitimate stall in progress. Yeah, I know it sounds stupid, but weight loss isn't a linear process, and our body weight fluctuates a lot day to day.

---

[*]*Starvation mode is often described as a physiological state where your body stores fat because you're not eating enough Calories. This is a complete myth, and you won't stop losing body fat if your Calorie intake is "too low"; it's physiologically impossible. If this were to happen, then contestants on TV survival programmes wouldn't lose any weight.*

This means that it may seem as though your weight loss has stalled, when really, it's just weight fluctuations masking your progress. So, you have to have at least 2 weeks minimum of consistently stalled readings to be sure it's a legitimate stall in progress.

Are You Being Honest With Yourself?

You have to be brutally honest with yourself here too:

- Have you been accurate in your food tracking, or are you eating mindlessly, and is your Calorie intake slowly creeping back up as a result? Common areas people miss are condiments, drinks (particularly hot ones with milk), fruit/veg, and the odd handful of cereal, nuts, or any other snack.

- Are you consistent with your training and activity level, or do you skip sessions, and opt for an evening of sofa sitting instead?

- Are you sticking to your plan pretty tightly throughout the whole week, or are you "cheating" hard and going out on the weekend, getting hammered, and stumbling home with a kebab, chips, and lemonade in your arms?

If you're not being consistent with your diet and training, then these areas need addressing before considering anything else, as it's likely nothing's wrong with your current plan; you just need to re-focus, hold yourself more accountable to your goal, and be consistent with it. Often, this re-focusing is all that's needed to get things going again, as it's human nature to get a little lax and creep back to old habits after dieting for a while.

While simply switching mental gears and re-focusing on your goal and plan may be all you need, you may have reached a point in your diet when it's time to metaphorically sit back, and relax by taking a diet break. This is something that – if programmed in periodically to your diet – can prevent such lapsing focus and motivation, and may ultimately steer you clear of road blocks in your progress.

DIET BREAKS CAN REBOOT YOUR MOTIVATION, DISCIPLINE, AND METABOLISM

Back in Chapter 3 when I discussed diet duration, I hinted that having a purposeful break from your diet could actually improve your results, and that by eating more during this period you could progress more effectively in the long run. The form of diet break I'm referring to here isn't an anything goes all out splurge on chocolate, sweets, or whatever else you've cut back on during your dieting; rather, it's a week or two where you bump your Calorie intake up to maintenance, and become less stringent with your tracking, while still retaining some level of control.

The purpose of such a diet break is twofold:

- **Psychological**

- **Physiological**

Allow me to explain …

The Benefits Of A Diet Break

Psychological

Anyone who's ever been on a diet for a significant amount of time will know that it takes its toll mentally. While many of the guidelines in previous chapters of this book should help minimise the mental impact dieting has on you, and make the process much easier, it is somewhat inevitable that you'll start to get fed up of dieting sooner or later. This can lead to waning motivation, more dietary slipups, and your Calorie intake starting to creep back up; no bueno.

A structured diet break can prevent this however, and by temporarily moving away from some of the constraints of dieting, and satisfying any cravings you have, you'll give your mental game a break. This means that come the end of the diet break, you'll have a renewed sense of discipline, fewer cravings, and a revival of motivation and focus.

Physiological

As detailed above, long periods of Calorie restriction come with their hormonal effects, and the associated knock on your metabolism. This can be reversed, to some extent, by bumping your Calorie intake back up for 1–2 weeks. Once you then return to your lower Calorie intake post break, you'll be in a strong position to continue your fat loss progress, which may occur at a faster rate due to your bolstered metabolism.

When To Have A Diet Break

I suggest you plan out when to have diet breaks before you get going with your shred. If your diet is 10 weeks long or less, then you probably won't need a break. However, if your diet is longer, then I suggest having a 1–2 week break every 10 weeks.

With that in mind, I've updated the diet duration table from Chapter 2.

Starting Body Fat %	Time To Reach 10%	Number Of Diet Breaks
11–13	3–6 weeks	0
14–16	8–12 weeks (+ diet breaks)	≤1
17–19	15–20 weeks (+ diet breaks)	1
20–24	20–30 weeks (+ diet breaks)	1–2
25–29	32–40 weeks (+ diet breaks)	2–3
30–35	>40 weeks (+ diet breaks)	≥3

Table 9.

How To Implement A Diet Break

There are the psychological and physiological aspects of the break to tackle here.

The **physiological** side will be covered by increasing your Calorie intake to your maintenance requirements. To do this, eat 20% more Calories by multiplying your current intake by 1.2. It is an increase in carbs – not fat or protein – that has the greatest benefits during your diet break, so get most of the extra Calories from carb sources. Because I suggest you don't track your macros when taking a diet break, you needn't worry about working out exactly how many extra carbs to consume; just be mindful to eat a couple of extra potatoes, slices of bread, or bowl of popcorn on top of your regular carb intake. If you've been using a portion control system during your diet, just add two more portions of carbs to each day's intake. As a result of

162

these extra Calories, your body weight might go up, particularly in the first few days of the break. If you're not going crazy with the Calories, this will simply be due to changes in water balance, and bodily carbohydrate stores. Gaining fat would require a larger increase in Calories to take your intake above maintenance levels. So don't stress if you follow these guidelines but end up gaining 1–2kg; it's not fat.

The **psychological** side of a diet break involves you being more laid back with the dietary management method you use; so take a step down on the precision ladder of management methods. For example, if you've been tracking your macros religiously for the last coupl'a months, track Calories only instead. If you've been using a portion control system, continue using that system, but with the extra carbohydrate portions.

What's important here is that you don't see your diet break as an excuse to pig out for a couple of weeks; you need to maintain a degree of control with your nutrition and fat loss plan, while taking a step back from the stresses of previous weeks of dieting. For this reason, it's important to stick to your regular meal patterns, weight training, and general daily structure.

So to summarise how to implement diet breaks:

- Have a 1–2 week diet break every 10 weeks of dieting.

- Increase your Calorie intake to maintenance.

- Favour more carbs as a means to increase your Calorie intake.

- Use a less demanding dietary management method.

- Maintain your regular meal patterns.

- Keep lifting as usual.

BREAKING THROUGH A PLATEAU

If you've planned in diet breaks, and have been consistent with your diet, yet your average weekly weight has legitimately stalled for at least a couple of weeks, then one way or another, you have to decrease the energy in and/or increase the energy outside of the equation, to create a Calorie deficit and kick things off again.

I suggest doing this in increments of 10%. By that, I mean create a 10% Calorie deficit by increasing expenditure and/or decreasing intake appropriately. If you're currently consuming 2300 Calories with no progress, that would mean adjusting by 230 Calories via increased expenditure, and/or decreased intake.

There are 3 main ways to go about doing this.

1. Add In Cardio

Give cardio a quick Google search and you'll be smacked in the face with all the online bickering over which form of cardio is best for fat loss. Ultimately, it depends on the context. For a detailed explanation as to why, visit the extra notes page on the bonus content area.

The main thing I want to drive home for now is that you view cardio in light of the bigger picture of Calories in vs Calories out (the "Fat Loss Switch", see Chapter 4). By that, I mean that cardio is primarily a means to burn Calories and help you achieve a Calorie deficit where your intake is less than your expenditure. So, the main thing to consider with your mode of cardio is to choose one that you enjoy and will stick to, be it high intensity, low intensity, cycling, running, or barbell complexes.

With that in mind, here are a few more guidelines to follow:

- Keep high intensity interval sessions to a max of 3 per week, as intense work will take more out of you and compromise recovery if you do too much (high intensity cardio will burn roughly 100–140 Calories per 10 minutes).

- Use low intensity cardio sessions (jogging, elliptical, cycling machine) as needed, to increase energy expenditure (you'll burn roughly 30–50 Calories per 10 minutes doing low intensity cardio).

- Start with the minimal effective dose, and taper up if needed. For example, you could start with 2x 20–30 minute cardio sessions a week. One might be a high intensity barbell complex session, and the other could be a low intensity bike ride. This would add up to around 300–400 extra Calories burnt in the week. You might then up this to a couple of longer low intensity sessions to burn more Calories without compromising recovery as greatly as high intensity cardio.

2. Increase Your NEAT And Step Count

Many don't realise that their activity level outside of the gym has a huge bearing on their results, and simply aiming to be more active in their day to day life can make a big difference and up Calorie burn significantly.

To do this, aim to hit a given step count each day (10,000 per day is a good starting point), and increase this if you need to burn more Calories. Although there are many factors dictating Calories burnt, and distance travelled per step:

2000 steps equate to roughly 100 Calories, and will take you a distance of one mile or so.

So you could add in a daily walk to bump up your step count by a few thousand, and consequently burn a couple hundred more Calories per day. I also suggest that you stand as frequently as possible (e.g. use a standing desk). While standing more won't necessarily kick start fat loss after a plateau, it is a very beneficial habit to get into.

3. Decrease Your Calorie Intake

If you choose to decrease your Calorie intake, then do so by reducing your carb and/or fat intake as opposed to protein. Whether you decrease carbs or fat should primarily come down to preference.

To do this, first take the number of Calories you want to drop and then divide it by 9 or 4, depending on whether you want to decrease fat or carb intake respectively. The result you get is the number of grams you need to drop your intake of each by. For example, if you want to decrease your intake by 200 Calories coming from carbs only, that's 50g of carbs (200 ÷ 4, as there are 4 Calories per gram of carbs).

Should You Increase Calorie Burn, Decrease Intake, Or A Combo Of The Two?

Whether you choose to re-ignite fat loss via more cardio, NEAT, and/or by decreasing your Calorie intake comes primarily down to your personal preference, and what you're more likely to adhere to.

Obviously, if your Calorie intake is already pretty low (e.g. circa 1600 Calories), then dropping it further will be a ball-ache; so in this scenario, you'd be best to introduce some cardio and/or NEAT to up your Calorie burn.

On the flipside, if you're already doing cardio and your Calorie intake isn't particularly low, then I'd suggest you drop Calorie intake.

In fact, if you're not entirely sure, and you're not eating a low Calorie, pigeon like, diet:

I advise you to go with dropping your daily Calorie intake by 10%.

This is for a few reasons:

- Changing Calorie intake is more reliable, as you may subconsciously change your day to day behaviour if you introduce more cardio. This is because your body may compensate for extra Calories burnt via cardio by moving less during other parts of the day.

- It's usually less of a pain in the arse to cut out a little food each day, compared to slogging out a couple of hours on a treadmill each week, as it takes quite some time/effort to burn Calories. Look back to the cardio example I gave above; for an hour's effort, you might burn in the region of 400 Calories, which you would have to do multiple times per week to get the job done.

- While doing an hour of Cardio might burn 400 Calories, you would have still burned Calories during that time if you hadn't done the exercise. For example, if you had sat on your arse drooling, while watching MasterChef for the hour instead, you would have burnt around 100 Calories in that time. So, that's a net extra Calorie burn of 300 from your hour of cardio. You need to take this difference into account, as it's the Calorie burn on top of what you usually do we're looking to increase.

Again though, you're the best judge of your personal preference and what you'll best adhere to, so it's your call on how you adjust things to create a 10% Calorie deficit.

Going back to our old friend, Ricky P as an example, let's say he has been spot on with his diet and training but his progress has stalled for 3 weeks. He's been eating 2000 Calories up until this point; so to re-ignite fat loss, he needs to alter this plan by 200 Calories (10%).

He could do this by:

- **Dropping Calorie intake:** Consuming 200 less Calories each day. That's just a cornetto's worth of food less per day, and adds up to 1400 fewer Calories over the week.

- **Increasing Calorie burn:** Burning 1400 more Calories per week from Cardio. That might be 3x one hour sessions of low intensity on the elliptical.

- **A combo of the two:** Consuming 100 fewer Calories per day, along with 2 extra cardio sessions per week.

Or, any other combo of upping Calorie burn, and decreasing intake.

Key Points

- Give at least 2 weeks of stalled progress before considering a change to your plan.

- A weight loss plateau may simply be due to waning adherence to your diet, which can be fixed by being honest with yourself and re-focusing on your goal and diet.

- As your diet progresses and you lose weight your metabolism/Calorie burn will drop to an extent; this is normal.

- The main causes of this lowered Calorie burn are a subconscious drop in movement/NEAT and the mere result of there being less of you to move about and burn Calories.

- If you've hit a plateau, you need to create a Calorie deficit of at least 10% by adjusting your intake or expenditure.

- Do this by increasing cardio, your step count, and/or by decreasing your Calorie intake from carbohydrate and fat. If you're not sure, simply decrease your daily Calorie intake by 10% and job's a good'un.

CHAPTER 13

How To Train When Dieting

While this book is nutrition focused, it would be remiss of me to neglect any mention of training, as developing a Herculean physique requires the duel force of both nutrition and training. So this chapter will quickly break down the foundations of training during a diet.

> I highly recommend you read my article titled "The Ultimate Training Programme For Building Muscle" (www.tommycole.co.uk/training-for-gains) and also my others on training which can be found at www.tommycole.co.uk/category/training.

HOW TO TRAIN WHEN DIETING

As discussed in Chapter 2, when dieting, gains in muscle are put on the backburner, and the main objective, from a muscle mass perspective, is to maintain as much as possible.

To explain how this is achieved with your training, you need to view your programme as a means to send signals to your body to encourage growth/muscle retention. So the exercises, number of reps, sets, and weight that you do all result in specific signals being sent to your muscles that dictate how your body responds. When your body receives these signals, it adapts accordingly.

This is why strength-oriented athletes, like the competitive strongman Hafthor Bjornsson (AKA: Gregor "The Mountain"),

171

train by lifting heavy weights, whereas endurance athletes, like Mo Farah, do low intensity and long duration training; their training is programmed in such a way that the signals it sends to their bodies cause them to adapt in a specific way (e.g. get bigger, stronger, more powerful, more efficient at burning energy, etc).

When it comes to dieting, the training that signals to your body to hold on to muscle is the same as that which causes your muscles to grow. That means:

Your training when dieting should be similar to when you're trying to gain muscle.

Which goes against what many believe, as it's often claimed that lighter weights and higher reps tone your muscles. In reality, what gives your body a toned look is losing body fat to reveal muscle:

- **Losing fat:** Losing body fat comes mostly down to your diet and what this book has covered up until now.

- **Revealing muscle:** As above, the aim of the game with muscle is to maintain it, which again will be greatly dictated by your diet, but your training has a big influence too.

So, the rest of this Chapter gives guidelines to follow in order to send the right signals to your body to achieve this. Again, you should read the articles I've linked above as they expand on this and provide example training programmes that apply all the key points.

I've also included an example intermediate lifter's training programme that applies all of the points.

TRAINING GUIDELINES WHEN DIETING

Volume (the amount of work you do per session): Each time you train a muscle group, do 4–8 sets in total. Start at the lower end if you're a beginner, and mid to upper if you're more experienced.

Intensity (the weight on the bar): You need to lift moderate to heavy weights to hold onto muscle. So, lift in the 6–12 rep range for the most part, going close to failure but only hitting absolute failure occasionally.

Frequency (the number of times you train): Train each muscle group more than once per week. 2–3 times per week is the sweet spot for most. In combo with the volume per session guideline above, this means a weekly volume of around 8–24 sets per muscle group. You should spread this training over 3–6 sessions per week.

Training split: This is how you organise your training sessions in the week. If you're training 3 times a week, I suggest 3 full body sessions as this will enable you to hit each muscle group 2–3 times in that week. An upper/lower split is better if you're training 4 times per week though (this works very well for beginners and intermediates), and for higher training frequencies you can split things up more (e.g. legs/push/pull). I recommend you read my article on training splits for more on this: www.tommycole.co.uk/best-training-split.

Exercises: For each muscle group you're training, you should do 1–3 compound exercises (ones that cause movement at more than one joint) as these will give you the most bang for your buck. Then add in 1–2 isolation exercises to get in the rest of your volume, and to zone in on any particular muscle you want to train. Below is a list of compound exercise examples to base most of your training on.

Movement	Main Muscles Worked	Exercise
Vertical pull	Back, biceps	Pull ups, chin ups, pull down.
Horizontal pull	Back, biceps	Bent over row, cable row, chest supported dumbbell row – you get the point; any variation of rows.
Vertical push	Shoulders, triceps	Variations of overhead pressing (dumbbell, barbell, half kneeling, etc).
Horizontal push	Chest, triceps, shoulders	Bench press, decline/incline bench press, dumbbell bench press variations, close grip bench, chest press, etc.
Quad dominant	Quadriceps, hamstrings, glutes	Back squat, front squats, split squats, lunge variations, leg press.
Hip dominant	Hamstrings, glutes, quadriceps	Deadlift, Romanian deadlift, barbell glute bridge.

Table 10.

Progression: While dramatic progress in your training is unlikely when dieting, you should still strive for progression if possible. To do this, incrementally increase the weight or number of reps/sets you're lifting over time. For example, add a rep or two, or 1–2kgs every other week. At the start of your diet you should be able to progress in this way, particularly if you're starting a new and improved training programme. As your diet goes on, your training progress may stall though, and you might have to slightly reduce the weight you're lifting, and/or volume. You're the best judge of this, so alter your training as and when required.

Example Training Programme

What follows is an example training programme that is based on 4 training sessions per week with an upper/lower split.

Session	Exercise	Sets	Reps
Session 1 (upper 1)	Bench Press	3	8–10
	Chest Supported Row	3	8–10
	Dumbbell Shoulder Press	3	8–10
	Pull Ups	3	10–12
	Close Grip Bench Press	3	10-12

Session	Exercise	Sets	Reps
Session 2 (lower 1)	Squat	3	8–10
	Deadlift	3	3–5
	Split Squat	3	8–10
	Hamstring curl	3	8–10
	Abs	2	1 min

Session	Exercise	Sets	Reps
Session 3 (upper 2)	Bench Press	3	4–6
	Bent Over Row	3	6–8
	Barbell Shoulder Press	3	6-8
	Lat Pull down	3	8–10
	Parallel Bar Dips	2	15–30

Session	Exercise	Sets	Reps
Session 4 (lower 2)	Squat	3	4–6
	Romanian Deadlift	3	8–10
	Leg Press	3	6–8
	Leg Extension	3	8–10
	Abs	2	1 min

Table 11.

Progression for the example programme: Start at the lower end of the rep range with a weight you can lift with 2–3 reps left in the tank on the first set. Once you can hit the lower end of the rep range for all sets with a given weight, add a rep next session (i.e. work up the rep range). Once you can hit the upper end of the rep range for all sets, add weight to the bar and start again at the lower end of the rep range. If you can't work up the rep range whilst maintaining good form, decrease the weight and start over.

CARDIO

As for cardio, it should be seen as a means to increase Calorie/energy expenditure as opposed to a direct trigger for fat loss. So, view it in light of the bigger picture which is creating a Calorie deficit.

Because the training you do signals to your body how to adapt, high amounts of cardio may hinder your physique related goals as your body has a finite ability to adapt. In other words, adaptations to cardio training compete with adaptations to your resistance training. This is why the strongest man in the world will never simultaneously be a marathon running champion, and is also why it's best to start with the minimal effective dose of cardio and then taper up if you need to rather than introducing lots from the off.

For cardio guidelines, shoot back to Chapter 12, and visit www.tommycole.co.uk/bookbonuscontent for a more in depth breakdown.

Key Points

- Training is a stimulus that your body adapts to by getting bigger, stronger etc.

- Resistance training when dieting should be relatively unchanged from a muscle gaining phase.

- The main factors to consider with your lifting are your training volume, intensity, split, exercises, and progression.

- Cardio should be seen as a means to increase Calorie/energy expenditure; not a direct cause of fat loss.

- Any cardio should be introduced with the minimal effective dose and tapered up if needed.

CHAPTER 14

The Diet After The Diet: Moving To Maintenance

Many guys who want a chiselled, athletic physique don't fail due to their inability to shred fat. No; the reason so many fail is because they struggle to keep it off post diet, as they find themselves returning to old habits and putting back on the weight they worked so hard to lose in the first place.

Much of this book has been working towards preventing this though:

- Incorporating your favourite foods to make your diet more enjoyable and sustainable.

- Teaching you how to find a dietary management method that suits you and your lifestyle.

- Expanding your nutrition knowledge.

And so on.

This means that once you reach your shredding goal, you won't be exhausted and fed up of eating a bland, overly restrictive, and rigid diet.

Where next though? Where should you go once you've finished your diet? And how should your plan of action change?

DO.NOT.WORRY. I've got your back, and will now cover what to do once you've finished dieting.

THE REVERSE DIET

The reverse diet is pretty self-explanatory, in that it's a process of flipping your diet upside down by increasing your Calorie intake to your maintenance needs.

There's a pervasive reverse dieting myth in the nutrition world that's spread about by many dieting Gurus though. What they suggest is that after your diet, you have to increase your Calorie intake very slowly (e.g. adding 50 Calories per week) to prevent fat re-gain, and that this gradual increase will actually cause you to continue losing fat while eating more Calories.

This is a floored idea though, primarily because regardless of how quickly you increase your food/Calorie intake to your maintenance level, you won't gain fat because you'll still be at or below your maintenance requirements. In other words, you won't have a surplus of Calories to store.

Kinda obvious when you think about it intuitively, right?

Continuing this line of thinking, when it comes to the persistent fat loss during a slow reverse diet, the only reason this happens is because you'll still be consuming a deficit of Calories until you reach maintenance; not because of any reverse dieting metabolic magic, as shown in Figure 32.

So, there really is no need to slowly increase Calories post diet, and the post diet goal is actually to get back to your maintenance needs, and a less restricted diet, as quickly as possible; this will help reverse the adaptations your body made to your diet, and enable you to have more dietary freedom faster.

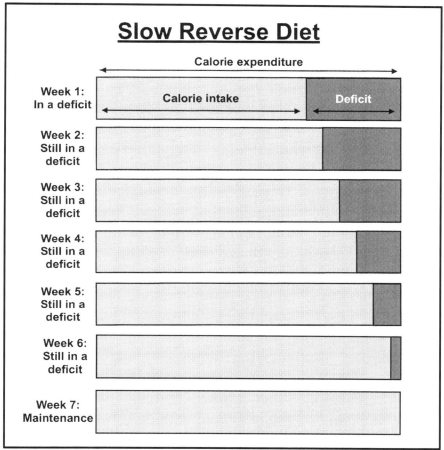

Figure 32.

HOW TO REVERSE DIET

The way you should approach your reverse diet is much like a diet break, in that you're:

1. Increasing your Calorie intake to get back to maintenance.

2. Moving towards a more laid back dietary management method.

I suggest you tackle these points in a step-like process. So focus on getting back to maintenance Calories first, and then consider your dietary management method after that.

Step 1: Increasing Calories To Maintenance

As above, this needn't be a long, drawn out process (unless you'd prefer it that way), and you can increase your Calories by around 20% from the off. I suggest starting with 300 extra Calories, which you should add mostly in the form of carbohydrates (e.g. 75g of carbs, or 50g of carbs and 11g of fat). The only caveat here is that you're adding these Calories to an intake that was causing you to lose weight at a rate of 0.5 kg per week or greater. If your weight loss had slowed to less than this, then add in fewer Calories.

Once you've added in Calories, stick to this intake for a couple of weeks and reassess how your body has responded to the added intake after this period. You may gain a kg or so, but if you haven't gone way overboard with Calories, this gain is nothing to worry about as it will be due to changes in water balance and your muscles filling up with carbs (this will actually make your physique look even better as your muscles will look fuller than they did during your diet).

You may continue to lose weight though. If this is the case, either the Calorie increase wasn't enough, or your body responded to the extra Calories by burning more (NEAT often goes up when you add in Calories post diet). To adjust from here, simply add 5% extra Calories every week until your weight stabilises and you reach maintenance needs.

Figure 33 is a visual representation of how the process works.

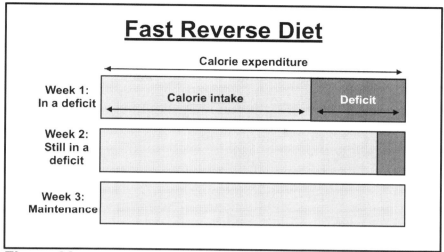

Figure 33.

This process of reaching your maintenance Calorie needs shouldn't take much longer than 2–3 weeks tops, and will set you in a good position to decide where you want to go next, while maintaining your level of leanness.

If you decide to then transition into a muscle gaining phase – which would require a further addition of Calories – then I advise you to stay at your maintenance intake for at least a couple of weeks first. This is because it will help reverse some of the adaptations your body made during your diet, and will prevent rapid fat gain from moving into a surplus of Calories too quickly; post diet your body is primed to gain fat, so if you move into a gaining phase straight away, you'll gain more fat than you would do if you take a couple of weeks at maintenance first.

Step 2: Moving Towards A More Laid Back Dietary Management Method

This takes us back to how The Big 3 dictate your dietary management method. Specifically, I'm referring to your Situation and where you are on your nutrition journey, which post diet, is a time where you'd probably like to figuratively, sit back and relax a little.

Now, I advise against relaxing too much here by easing off the dietary control all together, as you're prone to pigging out and regaining much of the fat you fought to lose. But, if you've been tracking macros tightly, then moving a step down the precision ladder of dietary management methods will relieve you of some of the stress that comes with dieting, without compromising your chiselled physique.

So, if you'd like, transition from tracking Calories and/or macros to tracking solely Calories, Calories and protein, or work towards implementing the portion control system.

If you do change dietary management methods, then I recommend you keep similar meal patterns and habits while you do so, as this will help you maintain control over your intake.

By following this measured, two-step process to your diet after the diet, you'll maintain the results you worked so hard for, and will be one of the few who don't relapse soon after reaching their goals.

Key Points

- Reverse dieting is a post diet process of increasing your Calorie intake to your maintenance needs.

- It's best to increase your Calorie intake back to your maintenance requirements as quickly as possible post diet.

- Unless your weight loss slowed to less than 0.5 kg per week at the end of your diet, increase your Calorie intake by 300 as the first step of your reverse diet. Favour an increase in carbohydrates as a means to add in these Calories.

- After 2 weeks, if your weight hasn't stabilized, this indicates that you haven't reached your maintenance requirements. So increase Calories by another 5% if this is the case.

- After your diet, I suggest you transition into a more laid back dietary management method.

- Don't ease off the dietary control all together.

- Maintain similar meal patterns and habits during your transition, as this will help you maintain control over your intake.

PART 6

THE ROUND UP

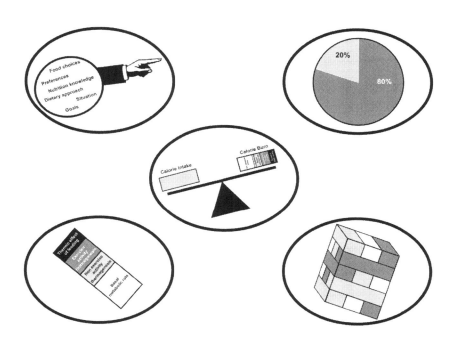

Chapter 15

The 10 Commandments Of The Smart Shred Diet

This chapter is here for my fellow brethren who have a goldfish-like attention span, and to give an extremely concise breakdown of the book's main recommendations.

Each commandment has a page number assigned to it, so use them as a reference point for the various topics of the book.

THE 10 COMMANDMENTS OF THE SMART SHRED DIET

1. Record your morning body weight 4+ times per week, and take progress pictures each week (pg. 21, 23).

2. Consume a deficit of Calories in order to lose 0.5–1% body weight per week. Use the calculations explained in Chapter 4 to work out your Calorie requirements (pg. 43).

3. Eat enough protein to maintain muscle, and to minimise hunger levels. Aim for around 2g per kg of target body weight (pg. 51).

4. The rest of your Calories come from carbs and fat. Make sure you eat enough carbs to fuel high intensity performance (pg. 69, 71).

5. Base your meal timing and frequency on your personal preference, and what you'll best adhere to. 3–6 meals per day, with each containing 30–50g of protein, will hit the sweet spot if you're looking to optimise results (pg. 52, 81).

6. Consider supplements if you've got the money to spend on them. Only a select few are beneficial, so refer to Chapter 8 for guidance (pg. 91).

7. Most of your diet (80% of Calories) should be made up of nutritious and minimally processed foods. Allow up to 20% of your Calories to come from whatever food you want though (pg. 113).

8. Follow the Smart Shred Diet System to dial in your diet. This science based system will ensure you shred body fat from the off, and ultimately attain a shredded physique with chiselled abs (pg. 137).

9. Have a 1–2 week diet break for every 10 weeks of dieting. During this break, increase your Calorie intake to maintenance (pg. 160).

10. Keep lifting heavy, walk at least 10,000 steps per day, and add in cardio if necessary to increase your Calorie burn (pg. 164, 171).

CHAPTER 16

The Debrief: Combining The "Smart" And The "Shred" To Transform Your Body

Pwoaaaa, that was muchos information you just read; so congrats. Seriously, well done for working your way through it all and getting to the end, as it has set you in a strong position for a successful Shred (I'd give you a cookie, but unfortunately Amazon don't give me that option as part of the whole Author package).

At this point, you're a fat loss ninja from a *"Smart"* perspective: You've advanced your nutrition knowledge to a level that puts you in the minority of people who genuinely know exactly how to lose fat and transform their body; most personal trainers don't even know the stuff you do.

Pretty sweet knowing that you're now in control of your body, and have the power to transform it and get ripped whenever you want, right?

It's now down to you to apply the *"Shred"* side of the equation by using what you've learnt throughout the book. All you have to do is follow the Smart Shred Diet System in Chapter 10 and be consistent with it. After just a few weeks you'll see noticeable changes in the mirror, and in 10–12 weeks your results will become more dramatic. Just visualise yourself at this stage and how you'll be thanking yourself for committing to your diet 12 weeks ago, as opposed to looking back and wishing you had started.

My goal with this book is to help you achieve that rippling, athletic body, but I can't do the hard work for you. So, like I promise that you'll see great results if you apply the information in this book, make a promise to both me and yourself that you'll commit to your Smart Shred Diet, and be consistent throughout the process. Take ownership of your body and diet; at the end of the day, you're the only one who can do anything about it.

I'd love to hear how you get on, so let me know at:

tommy@tommycole.co.uk

FINAL WORDS

Could You Do Me A Favour?

First off, thank you for buying this book; I hope you've enjoyed it, and I'm confident that if you apply what you've read, you'll be well on your way to a sculpted, lean, and athletic body.

Now we're at the end of the road, I have a favour to ask of you:

Would you mind sharing your thoughts and feedback of the book by giving it a review on Amazon?

A quick review will mean a hell of a lot, and I love to get feedback so I know that my work is helping people.

The following link will redirect you to the Amazon page where you can leave a review:

www.tommycole.co.uk/review

Also, if you have friends or fam who would enjoy and gain value from the book, be a bro by spreading the love and letting them borrow it.

Thanks again, and may your quest for cheese grater abs be Ben & Jerry like: smooth, enjoyable, and full of cookie dough (in moderation, of course).

Big love,

Tommy

12364288R00113

Printed in Great Britain
by Amazon